Environmental Health Criteria 104

PRINCIPLES FOR THE TOXICO-LOGICAL ASSESSMENT OF PESTICIDE RESIDUES IN FOOD

Published under the joint sponsorship of
the United Nations Environment Programme,
the International Labour Organisation,
and the World Health Organization

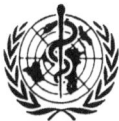

World Health Organization
Geneva, 1990

The **International Programme on Chemical Safety (IPCS)** is a joint venture of the United Nations Environment Programme, the International Labour Organisation, and the World Health Organization. The main objective of the IPCS is to carry out and disseminate evaluations of the effects of chemicals on human health and the quality of the environment. Supporting activities include the development of epidemiological, experimental laboratory, and risk-assessment methods that could produce internationally comparable results, and the development of manpower in the field of toxicology. Other activities carried out by the IPCS include the development of know-how for coping with chemical accidents, coordination of laboratory testing and epidemiological studies, and promotion of research on the mechanisms of the biological action of chemicals.

WHO Library Cataloguing in Publication Data

Principles for the toxicological assessment of pesticide residues
   in food.

(Environmental health criteria ; 104)

1. Pesticide residues - analysis - toxicity   2. Food contamination
I. Series

ISBN 92 4 157104 7   (NLM Classification: WA 240)
ISSN 0250-863X

Publications of the World Health Organization enjoy copyright protection in accordance with the provisions of Protocol 2 of the Universal Copyright Convention. For rights of reproduction or translation of WHO publications, in part or *in toto,* application should be made to the Office of Publications, World Health Organization, Geneva, Switzerland. The World Health Organization welcomes such applications.

The designations employed and the presentation of the material in this publication do not imply the expression of any opinion whatsoever on the part of the Secretariat of the World Health Organization concerning the legal status of any country, territory, city, or area or of its authorities, or concerning the delimitation of its frontiers or boundaries.

The mention of specific companies or of certain manufacturers' products does not imply that they are endorsed or recommended by the World Health Organization in preference to others of a similar nature that are not mentioned. Errors and omissions excepted, the names of proprietary products are distinguished by initial capital letters.

PRINTED IN FINLAND
89/8316 — VAMMALA — 5500
93/9570 — VAMMALA — 1000

CONTENTS

PRINCIPLES FOR THE TOXICOLOGICAL ASSESSMENT
OF PESTICIDE RESIDUES IN FOOD

FOREWORD   10

PREFACE   11

1. INTRODUCTION   13

2. GENERAL HISTORICAL BACKGROUND   15

3. JMPR ASSESSMENT PROCESS   17

4. CONSIDERATIONS OF IDENTITY, PURITY, AND STABILITY   21

    4.1 Background   21
    4.2 Principles   23
        4.2.1 Identity   23
        4.2.2 Purity   23
        4.2.3 Stability   23

5. AVAILABILITY AND QUALITY OF DATA   25

    5.1 Background   25
    5.2 Principles   26

6. HUMAN DATA   27

    6.1 Background   27
    6.2 Current position   28
    6.3 Principles   29

7. STRUCTURE-ACTIVITY RELATIONSHIPS   30

    7.1 Principle   30

8. TEST METHODOLOGIES   31

    8.1 Background   31
    8.2 General considerations   32
        8.2.1 Choice of species and strain   32
        8.2.2 Group size   33
        8.2.3 Selection of dose levels   36
        8.2.4 Test duration   38
        8.2.5 Pathological procedures   39
        8.2.6 Historical control data   40

8.3   Conduct and evaluation of studies   42
       8.3.1 Short- and long-term toxicity studies   42
       8.3.2 Carcinogenicity studies   47
              8.3.2.1 Background   48
              8.3.2.2 Routes of exposure   48
              8.3.2.3 Commonly occurring tumours   49
              8.3.2.4 Pathological classification of neoplasms   50
              8.3.2.5 Evaluation of carcinogenicity studies   51
              8.3.2.6 Extrapolation from animals to man   52
              8.3.2.7 Principles   53
       8.3.3 Reproduction studies   53
              8.3.3.1 Multigeneration reproduction studies   53
              8.3.3.2 Teratology studies   58
              8.3.3.3 Screening studies in teratology   60
              8.3.3.4 Principles   60
       8.3.4 Neurotoxicity studies   61
              8.3.4.1 Delayed neurotoxicity   61
              8.3.4.2 Acute neurotoxicity   63
              8.3.4.3 Chronic neurotoxicity   65
              8.3.4.4 Pyrethroid-induced neurotoxicity   65
              8.3.4.5 Neurobehavioural toxicity   66
              8.3.4.6 Principles   67
       8.3.5 Genotoxicity studies   67
              8.3.5.1 Principles   68
       8.3.6 Immunotoxicity studies   68
              8.3.6.1 Background   68
              8.3.6.2 Current position   69
              8.3.6.3 Principles   70
       8.3.7 Absorption, distribution, metabolism, and
              excretion   71
              8.3.7.1 Background   71
              8.3.7.2 Current position   72
              8.3.7.3 Principles   75

9.   EVALUATION OF DATA   76

     9.1 Extrapolation of animal data to humans   76
     9.2 Safety factors   76
          9.2.1 Background   76
          9.2.2 Principles   78
     9.3 Allocating the ADI   80
          9.3.1 Background   80
          9.3.2 Temporary ADIs   81
          9.3.3 Present position   82

10. EVALUATION OF MIXTURES   84

     10.1 Introduction   84
     10.2 Background   84
     10.3 Principle   84

11. RE-EVALUATION OF PESTICIDES   85

12. BIOTECHNOLOGY   86.

13. SPECIAL CONSIDERATIONS FOR INDIVIDUAL CLASSES
     OF PESTICIDES   87

     13.1 Organophosphates - ophthalmological effects   87
     13.2 Organophosphates - aliesterase (carboxylesterase)
           inhibition   87
     13.3 The need for carcinogenicity testing of
           organophosphates   88
     13.4 Ocular toxicity of bipyridilium compounds   88
     13.5 Goitrogenic carcinogens   88

REFERENCES   92

ANNEX I: GLOSSARY   109

ANNEX II: APPROXIMATE RELATION OF PARTS PER MILLION
          IN THE DIET TO MG/KG BODY WEIGHT PER DAY   113

INDEX   114

WHO TASK GROUP ON PRINCIPLES FOR THE TOXICOLOGICAL ASSESSMENT OF PESTICIDE RESIDUES IN FOOD

Dr N. Aldridge, The Robens Institute of Industrial & Environmental Health & Safety, University of Surrey, Guildford, Surrey, United Kingdom[a]

Dr G. Becking, International Programme on Chemical Safety, World Health Organization, Research Triangle Park, North Carolina, USA[a,e]

Professor C.L. Berry, Department of Morbid Anatomy, The London Hospital Medical College, London, United Kingdom[a,e]

Dr A.L. Black, Department of Community Services and Health, Woden, Australia[b,d,e]

Professor J.F. Borzelleca, Department of Pharmacology and Toxicology, Medical College of Virginia, Virginia Commonwealth University, Richmond, USA[d,e]

Dr G. Burin, Health Effects Division, Office of Pesticide Programs, US Environmental Protection Agency, Washington, DC, USA[b,c,e]

Dr J.R.P. Cabral, Unit of Mechanisms of Carcinogenesis, International Agency for Research on Cancer, Lyon, France[a]

Dr D.B. Clayson, Toxicology Research Division, Bureau of Chemical Safety, Food Directorate, Health and Welfare Canada, Ottawa, Ontario, Canada[e]

Mr D.J. Clegg, Agricultural Chemicals Section, Toxicological Evaluation Division, Food Directorate, Health Protection Branch, Ottawa, Canada[a,b,c,d,e]

Professor B. Goldstein, Rutgers Medical College, Busch Campus, Pescataway, New Jersey, USA[a]

Dr J.L. Herrman, International Programme on Chemical Safety, World Health Organization, Geneva, Switzerland[a,b,c]

Professor M. Ikeda, Department of Environmental Health, Tohoku University School of Medicine, Sendai, Japan[a]

Dr S.E. Jaggers, ICI Central Toxicology Laboratory, Cheshire, United Kingdom[e]

Dr F.-W. Kopisch-Obuch, Plant Protection Service, Food and Agriculture Organization, Rome, Italy[e]

Dr R. Kroes, National Institute of Public Health and Environmental Hygiene, Bilthoven, The Netherlands[a]

Professor M. Lotti, Istituto di Medicina del Lavoro, Università di Padova, Padova, Italy[a,b,d,e]

Dr L. Magos, Toxicology Unit, Medical Research Council Laboratories, Woodmansterne Road, Carshalton, Surrey, United Kingdom[a]

Dr K. Miller, Immunotoxicology Department, British Industrial Biological Research Association, Surrey, United Kingdom[e]

Professor R. Nilsson, The National Swedish Chemicals Inspectorate, Department for Scientific Documentation and Research, Solna, Sweden[e]

Dr A.K. Palmer, Reproductive Studies, Huntingdon Research Centre Ltd., Huntingdon, Cambridgeshire, United Kingdom[b,e]

Professor D.V. Parke, Department of Biochemistry, University of Surrey, Guildford, United Kingdom[a,e]

Dr O.E. Paynter, Health Effects Division, US Environmental Protection Agency, Washington, DC, USA[a,b,c,e]

Dr R. Plestina, Division of Vector Biology and Control, World Health Organization, Geneva, Switzerland[b]

Dr F.R. Puga, Section of Toxicology, Instituto Biològico, Sao Paulo, Brazil[d]

Professor A. Rico, Ecole Nationale Vétérinaire, Toulouse, France[e]

Dr L. Shuker, Unit of Carcinogen Identification and Evaluation, International Agency for Research on Cancer, Lyon, France[b,e]

Dr J. Steadman, Department of Health & Social Security, Hannibal House, Elephant and Castle, London, United Kingdom[a]

Dr E.M. den Tonkelaar, Toxicology Advisory Center, National Institute of Public Health and Environmental Protection, Bilthoven, The Netherlands[e]

Dr G. Ungvary, Section of Toxicology, National Institute of Occupational Health, Budapest, Hungary[d,e]

Dr G. Vettorazzi, International Toxicology Information Centre, San Sebastian, Spain[a,b,c,e]

NOTE TO READERS OF THE CRITERIA DOCUMENTS

Every effort has been made to present information in the criteria documents as accurately as possible without unduly delaying their publication. In the interest of all users of the environmental health criteria documents, readers are kindly requested to communicate any errors that may have occurred to the Manager of the International Programme on Chemical Safety, World Health Organization, Geneva, Switzerland, in order that they may be included in corrigenda, which will appear in subsequent volumes.

* * *

FOREWORD

The WHO activities concerned with the safety assessment of food chemicals were incorporated into the International Programme on Chemical Safety (IPCS) in 1980. These activities include administering the WHO Expert Group on Pesticide Residues, which meets regularly with the FAO Panel of Experts on Pesticide Residues in Food and the Environment in the well-known Joint FAO/WHO Meeting on Pesticide Residues, or JMPR. The objectives of the WHO Expert Group are consistent with those of IPCS, which include the formulation of "guiding principles for exposure limits, such as acceptable daily intakes for food additives and pesticide residues, and tolerances for toxic substances in food, air, water, soil, and the working environment." The inclusion of the present publication as a methodology document in the Environmental Health Criteria series will make it readily available to all of those who have an interest in the toxicological assessment of pesticide residues in food.

The IPCS gratefully acknowledges the financial and other support of the Canadian Health Protection Branch, the US Environmental Protection Agency, and the United Kingdom Department of Health. This support was indispensable for the completion of the project.

Dr M. Mercier
Manager
International Programme on
Chemical Safety

PREFACE

Since the early 1960s the Joint FAO/WHO Meeting on Pesticide Residues, usually known as the JMPR, has evaluated a large number of pesticides. The WHO component of these Joint Meetings, the WHO Expert Group on Pesticide Residues, has, during that time, relied upon procedures developed by other expert groups, such as the Joint FAO/WHO Expert Committee on Food Additives (JECFA), and developed specific principles for evaluating the various classes of pesticides that are used on food crops and may leave residues on them. The publication of WHO Environmental Health Criteria 70: Principles for the safety assessment of food additives and contaminants in food, which summarizes the assessment procedures used by JECFA, has been used by the WHO Expert Group on Pesticide Residues since its publication. Other principles specific to pesticides, however, have until now been scattered among the various JMPR reports, which has made it difficult for the WHO Expert Groups to use them in a consistent manner during their evaluations. In addition, many of the reports date back many years, and some of the advice given in earlier reports is no longer valid.

Recognizing the importance of maintaining consistency, an intercountry meeting that was held in 1985 in Ottawa, Ontario, Canada to consider ways of strengthening the role of JMPR in its evaluation of pesticide residues in food recommended that the principles that have been elaborated by JMPR through the years be codified and updated where appropriate and consolidated in a single publication. The 1985 JMPR supported such an effort and recommended "that this international meeting be requested to consider the toxicological basis and data requirements for the estimation of an ADI or temporary ADI, and to provide general guidance on relevant toxicological methodology."

An IPCS planning meeting was held in March 1987 in Carshalton, Surrey, UK in response to these recommendations, at which time areas were identified for consideration, which were incorporated into the first draft. This draft was reviewed at a task group meeting in Geneva in September 1988, after which extensive revisions were made. An editorial group meeting in Geneva in June 1989 produced the final draft, which was considered by the WHO Expert Group at the 1989 JMPR. Drafts were widely distributed at several stages, and the comments which were received from a wide range of international experts have been incorporated into the final publication.

The present publication therefore reflects the views of a large number of international experts who are involved with the toxicological assessment of pesticides. In addition, by concentrating on the procedures used by the WHO Expert Group on Pesticide Residues, it faithfully reflects the principles used in the evaluation of pesticide residues by JMPR. It is expected, therefore, that the future use of this publication by the WHO Expert Group will ensure consistent decision-making using up-to-date principles. Those involved in the production of this publication also hope that it will be of significant value to government officials responsible for establishing safe levels of pesticide residues on food commodities and by companies producing safety data on pesticides.

The WHO Expert Group on Pesticide Residues has been the responsibility of the International Programme on Chemical Safety (IPCS) since the inception of the Programme in 1980. The preparation of this publication provides an indication of the importance that IPCS places on the work of the WHO Expert Group in particular and on the toxicological assessment of pesticides in general. I am confident that those of us responsible for the toxicological assessment of pesticides will find the resources that have been put into the production of this publication to have been well-spent, and that the publication will be of enormous value in our work.

Dr J.L. Herrman
WHO Joint Secretary
Joint FAO/WHO Meeting on
Pesticide Residues

1. INTRODUCTION

The World Health Assembly noted in 1953 that the increasing use of various chemicals in the food industry had in recent decades created a new public health problem. In response to this, the World Health Organization, in conjunction with the Food and Agriculture Organization, initiated two series of annual meetings on food additives (Joint FAO/WHO Expert Committee on Food Additives, JECFA) and on pesticide residues. The first meeting on food additives was held in 1956 and that on pesticide residues in 1963.

Joint Meetings of the FAO Panel of Experts on Pesticide Residues in Food and the Environment and the WHO Expert Group on Pesticide Residues (usually referred to as the Joint FAO/WHO Meeting on Pesticide Residues, or JMPR) have provided an authoritative voice on the levels of pesticides that can be ingested daily by man without appreciable risk; this has been accomplished through the establishment of acceptable daily intakes (ADIs). Since 1966, JMPR has been establishing maximum residue limits (MRLs) of pesticides in food commodities.

This monograph has been prepared on behalf of the Central Unit of the International Programme on Chemical Safety (IPCS) and its aim is to provide an update of the principles utilized by the WHO Expert Group on Pesticide Residues. It does not address the work of the FAO Panel.

Certain toxicological principles pertinent to JMPR have previously been discussed in the JMPR reports. These principles usually relate to advances in scientific knowledge, which have modified both test procedures and the evaluation of test results. The contents of the JMPR reports were collated in 1977 [164]. Many of the basic principles were initially adopted from the deliberations of JECFA and are detailed in "Principles for the Safety Assessment of Food Additives and Contaminants in Food" [176]. In some of the areas where the principles used by JECFA and JMPR are identical, direct quotes from that publication have been included in this monograph. In this context, however, it should be recognized that the two committees, while utilizing data from similar types of studies, differ in their approach to the evaluation of the available data. This difference in approach arises because JECFA usually evaluates compounds intended for addition to food, which are usually of low toxic potential, whereas JMPR deals with residues of compounds that are toxic to at least some groups of living organisms.

The types of data that are evaluated when assessing the safety of a pesticide include those from biochemical and toxicological studies and, when available, observations in humans. The recent JMPR viewpoint is that an understanding of the pharmacokinetic and pharmacodynamic characteristics of a pesticide is extremely important and that such an understanding will even compensate for inadequacies in the available data base. On the other hand, this approach will sometimes lead to the requirement for either additional parameters to be investigated in routine studies or for additional specific studies not routinely required for the particular class of pesticide.

It has been recognized that data from studies using routes of exposure other than oral are of value in the overall evaluation of the safety of pesticides. However, these studies are not directly relevant for the calculation of the ADI, so this monograph will not consider these other routes of exposure in detail.

The more recent additions to the battery of toxicity tests available for use in safety assessment are discussed in this monograph. Some of these tests, especially in the fields of immunotoxicity and behavioural toxicity, are not yet at the stage of development where results are consistently reproducible and therefore readily utilizable in safety assessment. In addition, criteria for interpretation of such studies have not yet been sufficiently developed to be of value in routine safety assessment. Therefore, only the potential of these studies is discussed in this document.

The development of knowledge in the field of toxicology in recent years has been quite remarkable. The history of JMPR and the changes in its principles of safety assessment reflect this development. Thus decisions taken by JMPR are always provisional and ADIs are subject to re-evaluation as new significant data become available.

Each chapter in this monograph provides a rational background to a specific area, describes the history of relevant changes in principles according to the development of scientific knowledge, and offers a short summary of the current position of JMPR. It also indicates the principles being followed at present by the WHO Expert Group in their evaluations of pesticide residues in food and recommendations on how the studies may be performed to provide meaningful results.

2. GENERAL HISTORICAL BACKGROUND

The concept of JMPR was first proposed in 1959, when an FAO Panel of Experts on the Use of Pesticides in Agriculture [29], recommended that FAO and WHO should jointly study:

- the hazard to consumers arising from pesticide residues in and on food and feedstuffs;
- the establishment of principles governing the setting up of pesticide tolerances; and
- the feasibility of preparing an International Code for toxicological and residue data required in achieving the safe use of a pesticide.

Consequently, in 1961, a Joint Meeting of the FAO Panel of Experts on the Use of Pesticides in Agriculture and the WHO Expert Committee on Pesticide Residues was convened. The report of the 1961 Meeting [32] recommended to the Directors-General of FAO and of WHO the evaluation of "toxicological and other pertinent data . . . on those pesticides known to leave residues in food when used according to good agricultural practice". The evaluations would include the estimate of an acceptable daily intake and an explanation of its derivation.

To implement this recommendation the first Joint Meeting of the FAO Committee on Pesticide Residues in Agriculture and the WHO Expert Committee on Pesticide Residues was convened in September, 1963 [35]. This Meeting adopted the concept of the acceptable daily intake, which was based on:

- the chemical nature of the residue,
- the toxicity of the chemical based on data from acute, short-term, and long-term studies, and knowledge of metabolism, mechanism of action, and possible carcinogenicity of residue chemicals when consumed (usually determined in animals);
- knowledge of the effects of these chemicals on humans.

The 1963 JMPR [35] adopted the use of "safety factors" for extrapolating animal data to humans and to allow for variability within the human population. It also noted other points to be considered when establishing ADIs, including additive effects of multiple pesticides in the diet, potentiation between pesticide residues, and genetic differences (especially in enzyme composition) within the exposed human population.

The 1963 and 1965 Joint Meetings [35; 36] were concerned solely with the acceptable daily intake and did not consider tolerances. Separate meetings of an FAO Working Party on Pesticide Residues examined the issue of tolerances approximately two months after the Joint Meetings and issued separate reports. The first report considered principles [34] and the second proposed tolerances for pesticides on raw cereals [37].

In 1966, the JMPR report [38] considered both ADIs and tolerances for the first time. Joint Meetings have since been held yearly, and, after each one, reports and evaluations have been published. The JMPR has evolved principles consistent with the changing state of knowledge in toxicology and chemistry, and the evaluation of new data has often prompted adjustments in previous conclusions on various chemicals. However, the products of the Joint Meetings (which include ADIs, temporary ADIs, MRLs (MRL replacing the term "tolerance"), temporary MRLs, guideline levels, and extraneous residue limits) have remained essentially unchanged.

3. JMPR ASSESSMENT PROCESS

JMPR comprises two separate groups of scientists. The FAO Panel has responsibility for reviewing pesticide use patterns, data on the chemistry and composition of pesticides, and methods of analysis of pesticide residues, and for recommending MRLs that might occur in food commodities following the use of pesticides according to good agricultural practices. The WHO Group has responsibility for reviewing toxicological and related data and for estimating (where possible) an ADI for humans. During the Joint Meetings, the two groups coordinate activities and issue a joint report. However, the present section on interpretation of data is limited to the procedures used by the WHO Expert Group.

The data used in the assessment of the toxicity of pesticide residues generally comprise acute studies, short-term feeding studies, long-term feeding studies, and biochemical studies (including absorption, tissue distribution, excretion, metabolism, biological half-life, and effects on enzymes). In addition, studies on specific effects, e.g., carcinogenicity, reproduction, teratogenicity, and, for some compounds, neurotoxicity, are usually necessary. Human data and other information, e.g., SAR (structure-activity relationships), are also considered when available.

The overall objective of the evaluation is to determine a no-observed-adverse-effect level (NOAEL), based upon consideration of the total toxicology data base, which will be utilized in conjunction with an appropriate safety factor to determine the ADI. The initial stage of the evaluation has to be a critical examination of the individual studies. In some cases, a study initially considered to be of marginal value may, in fact, be useful when considered in the context of the entire data base. Integration of the results from all studies can then permit an appraisal of the toxicity of the compound.

Data from acute oral studies are rarely considered to be relevant to the establishment of the ADI. However, such data may provide information that permits a ranking of the sensitivity of different species, may assist in the selection of dose levels in subsequent studies, and may indicate types of pharmacological activity, degree of absorption, or potential target organs. JMPR has, on occasion, required additional acute data to determine the relative toxicity of salts of a pesticide (e.g., imazalil [57]) or required further metabolic studies to determine species differences in acute toxicity (e.g., triazophos [67]).

Historically, short-term feeding studies have provided the basis for the determination of ADIs for a number of compounds evaluated by JMPR. Prior to 1971 [48], before long-term toxicity studies were indicated to be an essential part of the toxicological data base for evaluating the safety of pesticides, ADIs were established for several pesticides based on short-term toxicity studies (e.g., demeton [45], parathion-methyl [182], dimethoate [182; 41], diazinon [182], azinphos-methyl [182], methyl bromide [39], and dichlorvos [39]). Temporary ADIs (TADIs) based on such studies have also been established, e.g., omethoate [49], fenthion [49]. Since long-term feeding studies have become an essential part of the toxicological data base, the major use of the data from short-term toxicity studies has been to determine suitable dose levels to be utilized in long-term and reproduction studies. However, studies lasting more than two years are rarely available in dogs. Thus, in situations where this species is more sensitive to a toxic effect or more appropriate for use in extrapolation to humans than are the rodent species, the ADI is usually based on data generated in studies covering less than 50% of the lifespan of this species, e.g., methamidophos [182], diflubenzuron [182], and phenthoate [63; 73]. Occasionally, an ADI may also be based on short-term studies in rodent species, e.g., diphenylamine [56; 68; 73], even though long-term studies may exist which indicate higher NOAELs. This situation may arise from adaptation, resulting in the disappearance of an effect after long-term exposure.

Multigeneration reproduction and teratogenicity studies have also been used for establishing ADIs for certain compounds, e.g., chlormequat [51] and dinocap [183].

Delayed neurotoxicity has been identified as a potential problem for a number of compounds evaluated by JMPR. To date, only leptophos has had an ADI withdrawn because of this effect. However, withdrawal of the ADI was not because of possible hazards from exposure to food residues but because of withdrawal of the product from the market as a result of effects on heavily exposed individuals during its manufacture [59]. ADIs have been allocated for other delayed neurotoxicants, e.g., isofenphos [76]. JMPR has indicated that the exaggerated doses (exceeding the LD_{50}) used in the standard hen studies for delayed neurotoxicity are not necessarily applicable to the assessment of human hazard arising from the intake of residues in food.

For the effects discussed above, the basic interpretation of the available data depends upon the identification of a toxic effect, the establishment of incremental increases in the incidence of this effect with increasing exposure (i.e. a dose-effect relationship), and the establishment of a threshold.

The primary consideration in determining whether a compound can induce a toxic effect is the dose of test material to which the test organism is exposed. A basic concept of toxicology is the statement made by Paracelsus in 1538, which translated indicates: "Only the dose decides that a thing is not poisonous" [1]. Thus, if a series of doses used in a study fails to elicit a toxic response, then an insufficiently high dose level has been used. This philosophy is applicable to all toxicity studies. However, provided an adequate margin of safety exists between the highest dose tested and the possible human exposure from pesticide residues, then a study in which a toxic effect was not observed may be considered to be acceptable for the purpose of assessing the safety of such residues. The major difficulty in the absence of toxicity is the determination of the safety factor to be applied to the highest dose tested, since there would be no indication of the type, importance, or severity of the effect that might be induced with increased dose levels.

A second factor is the determination of which effects should be considered to be toxic. A judgment must be made, based on the nature of the effect, on whether it should be considered adverse. As indicated in section 8.3.6.2, plasma cholinesterase depression should not be considered to be a toxic phenomenon since, although it is an effect, it is not apparently a *toxic* effect. A reversible increase in liver weight may be an adaptive response rather than a toxic effect. However, ancillary studies may be required.

The determination of dose-response relationships in an experimental population is based on the concept that the incidence or severity of an adverse effect is related to dose. A time-response relationship may also occur, i.e. where the incidence of an induced effect increases with the duration of dosing at a constant level. Comparison of the results of experiments with differing durations (performed on the same species and strain, preferably in the same laboratory, and under similar environmental conditions) may be necessary to demonstrate time-effect relationships if interim kills have not been performed. In the absence of interim kills or shorter-term experiments for comparative examination, it is sometimes possible to calculate the approximate time of appearance of a major lesion based on findings in dying animals or those sacrificed in moribund condition during the course of the study, particularly if the lesion is associated with the cause of death.

The integrated nature of mammalian reproductive processes may complicate the establishment of dose/time/response relationships for reproductive effects. Events that are initiated during early development may be moderated considerably in subsequent developmental stages. The defense mechanisms which have evolved to minimize the consequences of insult may repair minimal damage or discard that which is damaged beyond effective repair (e.g., resorptions or abortions). Consequently, in reproduction studies, the demonstrated dose response is often a reflection of a progressive involvement of multiple variables rather than a temporal change in a single variable.

When evaluating toxicological data, relevant parameters are evaluated statistically so that their significance is established on the basis of predetermined criteria. A statistically significant difference between experimental and control groups should be considered in the light of its biological relevance. Thus, an increased incidence of a rare tumour type in treated animals may be of concern, even if the incidence is not significantly different statistically from its incidence in the concurrent control animals. Conversely, a statistically significant change in an isolated parameter, e.g., erythrocyte count, would usually not be considered to be biologically relevant unless supported by changes in other parameters, e.g., bone marrow or spleen histopathology or methaemoglobin formation.

A high background incidence of a specific lesion frequently complicates the interpretation of data generated in toxicity studies. To some extent, especially in the case of a specific tumour type, this problem can be avoided by judicious choice of species or strains of animals. For example, if the target organ is known to be the kidney, the interpretation of results would be difficult in long-term studies in a rat strain with a high incidence of geriatric nephropathy.

The use of more than one species for the same type of toxicity study may complicate interpretation in those cases where an effect occurs in one species but not in a second species, or where one species is much more sensitive to the agent than the other species. In such cases it is often difficult to determine the most appropriate species for extrapolation to man. Generally, unless adequate data are available to indicate the most appropriate species (usually comparative pharmaco-kinetic or pharmacodynamic data), the most sensitive species (i.e., the species in which the adverse effect occurred at the lower dose) is used in determining the NOAEL and allocating the ADI.

In interpreting carcinogenicity data, JMPR bases its evaluations on the threshold concept, which is the basis for evaluating most other toxicological effects [170]. In assessing tumour incidence, benign and malignant tumours have been considered as separate entities in the majority of cases [176]. For further discussion of the determination of NOAELs in carcinogenicity studies, see section 8.3.4.5.

The 1986 Joint Meeting stressed the importance of understanding the mechanism of action that results in the expression of toxicity. It noted that: "Current knowledge of mechanisms of toxicity is limited, but there is already a sufficient understanding in some cases to permit better design, performance, and interpretation of toxicological studies. Mechanistic studies are therefore encouraged, since a knowl-edge of mechanism of action is likely to result in a more rational assessment of the risk to man." [76, p. 2].

4. CONSIDERATIONS OF IDENTITY, PURITY, AND STABILITY

4.1 Background

The report of the WHO Scientific Group on Procedures for Investigating Intentional and Unintentional Food Additives indicated in 1967 that: "adequate specifications for identity and purity should be available before toxicological work is initiated. Toxicologists and regulatory bodies need assurance that the material to be tested corresponds to that to be used in practice." It also stated that: "levels of impurities that, according to current knowledge, are considered to be toxicologically significant . . . must appear in the specifications." [169, p. 8].

The need for accurate specifications for pesticides was stressed by the 1968 JMPR [42] during its deliberations on toxaphene and on technical grades of benzene hexachloride (BHC). Because of the unknown or variable composition of these compounds, the JMPR was unable to relate the existing toxicological data to the products in actual agricultural use. Consequently, ADIs could not be allocated. Attention was also drawn to the likelihood of variability between similar chemicals produced by different manufacturers.

The possible influence of known or unknown impurities on the toxicity of technical grade chemicals and of residues resulting from their use was discussed by the 1974 JMPR [53]. This JMPR noted that toxicity studies are generally performed on technical grade materials produced by commercial-scale processes and that the resulting toxicological data normally, therefore, take into account the presence of impurities (provided that the manufacturing process remains the same). However, it noted the problems encountered with trace amounts of biologically active materials, e.g., 2,3,7,8-tetrachloro-dibenzo-p-dioxin in 2,4,5-trichloroacetic acid. It further noted that: "specifications such as those issued by FAO and WHO are seldom designed to take note of trace-level impurities, unless the importance of such impurities has already been revealed by biological studies." [53, p. 15].

The 1977 JMPR [57] noted that data on the nature and level of impurities, intermediates, and by-products in technical pesticides were often available, but, because such data could provide valuable information to competitors they were normally considered to be a "trade secret". The Joint Meeting, therefore, agreed that such data would not normally be published in the JMPR reports or monographs.

In considering the applicability of recommendations to pesticides from different feedstocks produced by different manufacturers, the 1978 JMPR [59] indicated that evaluations and recommendations are valid only for the specific technical grade of pesticide examined. Considerable care and knowledge of the detailed specifications are required to extrapolate evaluations and recommendations to products of differing quality or composition.

Subsequent Joint Meetings [60; 62; 72] have stressed the importance of information on the presence of impurities in technical pesticide products (e.g., the presence of hexachlorobenzene in various pesticides, impurities in phenthoate, and dimethyl hydrazine in maleic hydrazide). The need for technical grade pesticides to meet FAO specifications has also been stressed. It was noted by the 1984 JMPR that occasionally data have been rejected because the test material failed to comply with these specifications [72].

The 1987 JMPR [78] noted that ADIs based on studies using compounds of specific purity can be relevant to products of different origin or purity but that there are examples of changes in the amount or type of impurity in the technical material that markedly influence the toxicity of a compound.

Toxicity tests should normally be performed on the technical grade of the pesticide (except for acute toxicity, for which both formulations and technical materials must be tested to assess the risk to the applicator). However, the percentage of active ingredient and impurities in the technical grade material may vary among production batches and may differ at various stages of product development. Furthermore, since some toxicity testing is likely to be performed with the product in the early stages of development, the preliminary studies (usually designed to assess potential acute hazards to individuals who will be involved in the development of the material) may be performed on batches of material produced within the laboratory. Subsequent studies may be performed on material produced in a pilot plant, while other toxicity studies may be performed on the marketed product, which will be produced in a full-scale manufacturing plant. At each step in this sequence, there is a potential for change in the percentage of the active ingredient in the "technical-grade" material and a potential for change in the quantity and identity of the impurities that constitute the remainder of the "technical-grade" product. It is, therefore, essential that detailed specifications should be provided for the test material utilized in each study.

In certain cases the pesticidally active ingredient may exist in two or more forms, e.g., as a diastereoisomeric mixture. In the case of the synthetic pyrethroids, this is normally the case. Under such conditions, the ratio of isomers in the test material must be clearly specified since it has been documented that different isomers frequently have different toxicological activities [60; 87]. For example, an ADI for permethrin (40% cis : 60% trans) was allocated in 1982 [67], whereas the ADI for permethrin (25% cis : 75% trans) was not allocated until 1987 [78].

Data on the stability of the test material is also of importance. The percentage of the active material will decrease and that of breakdown products will increase with time if a test compound is unstable under the conditions of storage. This will be of major importance in the evaluation of the results of studies where a single batch of technical material is utilized for a long-term study or a multigeneration study. Variation in the amount of degradation occurring in different

batches (i.e., batches of different post-manufacturing age) may complicate the interpretation of a study. Finally, reaction of the test
compound with components of the test diet may result in the production
of toxic reaction products in the diet, which may affect the nutritive
value of the diet and will result in a decreased concentration of test
compound. The NOAEL may well be overestimated if the percentage of
active ingredient decreases with time. Conversely, if a breakdown
product is more toxic than the parent active material, then the NOAEL
of the parent compound may be underestimated. Either situation would
result in the establishment of an inaccurate ADI.

Up to now, JMPR has evaluated only the active ingredients of pesticide formulations. The toxicity of "inert ingredients" (e.g., sol-
vents, emulsifiers, preservatives) that may occur as residues in food
has not been considered.

4.2 Principles

4.2.1   Identity

(a) A detailed specification of the test material used in each individual study must be provided.

(b) Where isomeric mixtures exist, the ratio of isomers in the test
material must be clearly specified, since it has been amply documented that different isomers frequently have different toxicological activities.

(c) JMPR recommendations relate to a specific technical grade of a
pesticide. They will not necessarily be applicable to similar
materials produced by different manufacturers or where specifications of new material used in the manufacturing process are not
consistent.

4.2.2   Purity

(a) The percentage of the active ingredient in any technical material
used in a toxicity test or proposed for marketing must be specified.

(b) Levels of all identifiable impurities should be specified.

(c) Data on manufacturing processes may be required to permit determination of potential impurities. However, because of confidentiality
and industrial secrecy, such data will not be published in JMPR
monographs.

4.2.3   Stability

(a) Stability of the test material during storage and in the diet must
be adequately investigated and reported.

(b) Where instability in diets is observed, possible reaction products and the nutritional quality of the diet should be investigated.

5. AVAILABILITY AND QUALITY OF DATA

5.1 Background

Most of the data utilized by JMPR consists of unpublished pro-prietary data, as well as information submitted by governments and other interested parties. When available, relevant reports from the open literature are considered. However, published data on major studies must provide sufficient information to permit evaluation [38; 57]. This precludes reliance on summary or abstract publications. Such information must include complete descriptions of experimental tech-niques and data adequate to permit assessment of the validity of the results [38]. It is preferable that published reports be from refereed journals. Although all available relevant data are considered [46; 54], unpublished data must meet certain criteria, i.e. reports must be complete, study supervisors should be qualified to perform the study and should be identified, and the time at which the study was performed must be identified [38; 46].

Only those data which are available to all members can be con-sidered during a Joint Meeting [55]. This requirement applies to all supporting data and cited material. This has been a subject of ongoing concern and has been addressed frequently in JMPR reports [53; 54; 55; 57; 59; 60; 62; 65; 67; 70; 78; 172].

On some occasions, important information is omitted from the report of a study. Examples of such information include the identity and specifications of test material (section 4), information on the quality of experimental animal diets, and information on their nutritional composition.

Present-day standards generally require that data should be subject to quality control and that the study should conform to the standards specified under codes of good laboratory practice (GLP) [160; 161]. Studies performed in compliance with GLP codes help assure that the quality of unpublished data is acceptable. However, compliance with GLP codes does not provide a substitute for scientific quality. An inappro-priate study is still unacceptable even though it may have been con-ducted according to GLP standards.

The validity of data submitted for evaluation has always been of concern. Recent scandals reported in the scientific literature, in-volving inaccurate or falsified data [12], highlight this problem of data validity. However, the application of "good laboratory practice" and "quality assurance" techniques should reduce, but probably will not eliminate, the problems of data validation.

JMPR does not have the resources to validate studies [59]. There-fore, it accepts submitted data as being valid unless there is evidence to the contrary [57]. The 1977 JMPR [57] was informed of the suspicion that serious deficiencies existed in several studies that had been utilized by JMPR in allocating some ADIs and TADIs. In 1982, the Meeting re-evaluated a number of pesticides that had been supported by data from Industrial Bio-Test Laboratories. As a general principle, where studies supporting the ADI could not be validated, and where alternative studies were unavailable, the ADI was converted to a temporary ADI. Furthermore, if the studies were not validated or replaced, the ADI was withdrawn.

The format for data presentation requires that a summary of all pertinent studies be prepared [57], together with reports of each study with complete supporting data. Complete supporting data are usually considered to be individual animal data, although occasionally, if GLP codes have been followed and quality control assurance is available, this requirement has been waived. The submission of an evaluation of the compound by the sponsor is encouraged. Since the working language of JMPR is English [65], translations of reports into English are appreciated.

5.2 Principles

1. To evaluate the safety of pesticide residues, JMPR is dependent upon the receipt of acceptable data. Data for major studies should not be in abstract or summary format and should be of good scientific quality from laboratories utilizing acceptable laboratory practices [46; 54; 57; 59; 60; 62].

2. Compliance with recognized GLP codes (e.g., those of OECD) is encouraged.

3. Submitted data should be in such a form that the integrity of the study can be ascertained.

6. HUMAN DATA

6.1 Background

Human data on pesticides are collected from a variety of sources including accidental, occupational, and experimental exposures. Data from experimental exposures of human volunteers can provide quantitative information on dose-effect and dose-response relationships which may be applied directly in establishing an ADI. Data on accidental and occupational exposure can serve as supporting information.

A Joint FAO/WHO Meeting in 1961 highlighted the relevance of human data for toxicological evaluations and the need to study occupational exposures during production, handling, and uses of pesticides, since exposure is generally higher than that of the general population [32].

In 1967, a WHO Scientific Group was convened to provide guidance for the review of intentional and unintentional food additives. This group addressed the general problem of investigations in human subjects and recommended the conduct of human metabolic studies. It was recognized that adequate preliminary tests in animals are necessary before *in vivo* human studies can be performed [169]. In addition, studies in volunteers might be required to confirm the predicted safety margin. However, several conditions were listed which should be fulfilled before such studies can be undertaken, including the demonstration of need and full information on toxicity in experimental animals and the reversibility of toxic effects. The Scientific Group indicated that experimental studies on the toxic effects of pesticides in humans are not acceptable.

At the 1968 and 1969 Joint Meetings [42; 44], it was stated that the availability of adequate human data might justify the use of lower safety factors in setting the ADI [46].

The use of modern quantitative analytical toxicology concepts was introduced at the 1973 JMPR [52], with suggestions of the analysis of tissue and body fluids for a given pesticide. This is of particular importance in accidental poisonings. This Joint Meeting also suggested the follow-up of workers exposed to pesticides. Observations in such studies may reveal effects specific to humans. The 1975 Joint Meeting recommended to WHO that cooperation should be sought with Poison Control Centres and other organizations to develop appropriate data banks [54].

Data from humans continued to be required in relation to a number of pesticides until the time of the 1976 JMPR [55]. After that time, because of ethical problems and the increasing difficulties of performing studies in humans, JMPR reports indicated that data on humans were "desirable". Since 1982 [67], JMPR has generally, when toxicological assessments have been performed, indicated the desirability of data on observations in humans. When considering again the need for comparative biotransformation data, the 1987 JMPR [62] stated that these might also be obtained with *in vitro* experiments. It should be noted that there are limitations in the use of *in vitro* data, in that absorption and subsequent distribution as well as possible activation mechanisms must be considered before extrapolating such data to the *in vivo* situation and the subsequent establishment of an ADI.

The 1989 JMPR re-emphasized the necessity of obtaining human data. It indicated that human data may confirm a common mechanism of toxicity between humans and the test species or may be used to compare doses and effects between species [183].

6.2 Current Position

All human data (accidental, occupational, and experimental exposures) are fundamental for the overall toxicological evaluation of pesticides and their residues in food. Data on accidental poisonings may identify target organs, dose-effect and dose-response relationships, and the reversibility of toxic effects, provided that modern standards of analytical toxicology (e.g., identity and purity of the pesticide, blood levels of the parent compound and/or breakdown products, gastric lavage content, and urinary metabolites) have been applied to the study. A careful assessment of the dose and perhaps of the effects (e.g., plasma and erythrocyte cholinesterase inhibition) may enable comparison with animal data. Unfortunately, available data rarely permit such comparison. Follow-up studies in workers may enable the validity of extrapolations from animal data to humans to be confirmed and unexpected adverse effects specific to humans to be detected.

The JMPR mandate is to consider the safety of pesticide residues in food. Dietary exposure on a daily basis is almost always relatively low compared to occupational exposure, and therefore it might be expected that an effect on the exposed worker would be more easily detected. Unfortunately, there are limitations in attempting to extrapolate observations in the occupational setting to dietary exposure. The major route of exposure to pesticides for workers is generally dermal. The extent and rate of absorption via the dermal route usually differs markedly from that observed after oral exposure. Ingested compounds may be metabolized by intestinal microflora and may be subject to metabolism within the liver directly after absorption from the gastrointestinal tract and transport by the hepatic portal system. Thus target tissues may be exposed to a different pattern of parent compound and metabolites after dermal or inhalation administration than after oral administration. Data on the identity and levels of parent compound and metabolite(s), following administration by the different routes, are desirable to assist in the interpretation of the observed toxic effects.

When large groups of individuals are exposed to pesticides, epidemiological studies can be of considerable value. Often, however, workers in manufacturing plants and pesticide mixer/loaders and applicators are also exposed to several other compounds and it may be difficult to determine a cause-effect relationship for a given pesticide.

Results are also often confounded by the difficulty in finding suitable control populations, the large number of other variables involved, the long latency period for certain effects such as cancer, and small study populations, especially in manufacturing facilities. Exposure levels may also be difficult to quantify. Further guidance in the conduct and interpretation of epidemiological studies is given in Environmental Health Criteria 27 [173].

Studies on human volunteers are sometimes of considerable value in allocating ADIs. However, before human *in vivo* studies are considered, ethical considerations must be taken into account. The Proposed Guidelines on Biomedical Research Involving Human Subjects, issued as a joint project by WHO and the Council for International Organizations of Medical Sciences [21], have been endorsed by JMPR.

The value of human data was expressed cogently by Paget [127], when he wrote:

"The question is not whether or not human subjects should be used in toxicity experiments but rather whether such chemicals, deemed from animal toxicity studies to be relatively safe, should be released first to controlled, carefully monitored groups of human subjects, instead of being released indiscriminately to large populations with no monitoring and with little or no opportunity to observe adverse effects."

6.3 Principles

1. The submission of human data, with the aim of establishing dose-effect and dose-response relationships in humans, is strongly encouraged.

2. Studies on volunteers are of key relevance for extrapolating animal data to humans. However, attention to ethical issues is necessary.

3. The use of comparative metabolic data between humans and other animal species for the purpose of extrapolation is recommended.

7. STRUCTURE-ACTIVITY RELATIONSHIPS

The Joint FAO/WHO Meeting on Principles Governing Consumer Safety in Relation to Pesticide Residues recognized that toxicological "procedures must be determined by the chemical and physical properties of the pesticide . . . " [1, p. 8]. A subsequent WHO Scientific Group stated that: "If a series of chemical analogues can be shown to give rise to the same main metabolic product and other compounds which are already present in the organism in greater quantities, or that can be readily and safely metabolized, it may be sufficient to carry out toxicological studies on a suitable representative of the series." [169, p. 7]. The same Meeting, in considering the duration of studies, also indicated that: "Where adequate biochemical and toxicological data on closely related compounds are available, the objective becomes the detection of any deviation from the established pattern" [169, p. 13]. This latter principle has been exemplified by some evaluations of dithiocarbamate pesticides, where related compounds were considered as a group.

Structure-activity considerations can influence the testing needs of a pesticide. Thus the organophosphorus compounds, especially those with the P-S configuration, are routinely tested for delayed neurotoxicity, while the majority of other pesticides are not. Similarly, neurotoxicity is carefully considered in assessing the safety of the synthetic pyrethroid compounds.

The limitations of the use of structure-activity relationships has been discussed in the recent document on Principles for the Assessment of Food Additives and Contaminants in Food:

"Structure-activity relationships appear to provide a reasonably good basis for predicting toxicity for some categories of compounds, primarily carcinogens, which are characterized by specific functional groups (e.g., nitrosamines, carbamates, epoxides, and aromatic amines) or by structural features and specific atomic arrangements (e.g., polycyclic aromatic hydrocarbons and aflatoxins). However, all these chemical groups have some members that do not seem to be carcinogenic or are only weakly so." [176, p. 27-28].

For detailed information on the various chemical classes associated with carcinogenesis, the reader is referred to published review articles [146; 178].

7.1 Principle

For the determination of ADIs, JMPR relies primarily on data generated on individual chemicals. Structure-activity considerations are used only as ancillary information.

8. TEST METHODOLOGIES

The design and conduct of toxicological investigations has always been, and still remains, the responsibility of competent experts in the field. Therefore, the following sections and subsections should be considered only as guidelines unless stated otherwise.

8.1 Background

The second and fifth reports of JECFA addressed the conduct and uses of acute, short-term, long-term, biochemical, and carcinogenicity studies in the safety evaluation of food additives [31; 33]. While many of the proposals included in these documents have changed with advancing knowledge in toxicology, some are still deemed to be valid. These include:

- the need for short-term studies in rodents and non-rodents (defined as studies comprising repeated doses over a period of up to 10% of the expected lifespan of the animal, i.e., usually 90 days in rats and 1 year in dogs);

- the non-requirement for determining LD_{50} values when no mortality occurs at doses of 5 g/kg body weight or more;

- the need to initiate short- and long-term studies in young (post-weaning) animals;

- the need for uniform distribution of the test compound in the diet when feeding studies are utilized;

- the requirement to use *both* sexes in acute, short-term, long-term (chronic), and carcinogenicity studies;

- the need for initiating studies with sufficient animals to ensure adequate numbers of survivors to provide data for proper statistical analysis;

- the need to restrict the amount of test compound to less than 10% of the diet when performing feeding studies (although today it is generally recommended not to exceed a dietary level of 1% for a pesticide);

- the need, on a routine basis, for data on absorption, distribution, and excretion, and, where possible, identification of the major metabolites;

- investigation of the effects of dose level and duration on the metabolism of the test material;

• the need to test contaminants in food for carcinogenicity by oral administration;

• the requirement to maintain an adequate nutritional status of the test animal in feeding studies, especially in carcinogenicity studies. Information on the quality and composition of the diets used in toxicology studies should be provided.

The first JMPR [35] indicated that the biological data required for allocation of an ADI should include biochemical, acute, short-term (defined as repeated administration for less than half the lifespan), and long-term studies. The 1976 JMPR outlined the data necessary for the evaluation of pesticides. These included short- and long-term studies, special studies on carcinogenicity, mutagenicity, reproduction, and teratology, observations in humans, and information on metabolism, pharmacokinetics, and biochemical effects [55, p. 8-9]. These are the studies that are now generally available for pesticides used on food items. Salient aspects of the toxicological tests most often used in determining the safety of pesticide residues in food are discussed in the following sections.

8.2 General Considerations

8.2.1 Choice of species and strain

Limitations are inherent in the selection of laboratory animal species. The most readily available test species are the rat, mouse, hamster, guinea-pig, rabbit, cat, dog, pig, and monkey. More exotic animals (e.g., Tupia) are also utilized but only rarely. The major reasons for the use of such a limited number of species include economics (cost of obtaining and maintaining animals), lifespan, behaviour and survival in captivity, handling, and, perhaps most importantly, knowledge of the "normal" physiology and pathology of the species (see section 8.2.6).

In 1967, a WHO Scientific Group indicated the need to utilize the most appropriate species in extrapolating to man, i.e., "the species most similar to man with regard to its metabolic, biochemical, and toxicological characteristics in relation to the subject under test" [169, p. 9]. The choice of an ideal test species requires considerable knowledge of the absorption and biotransformation of the test material, not only in the experimental animal species, but also in humans. Unfortunately, other considerations (e.g., cost or availability of test species, duration of the study) must also be considered, and it is not always practical to use the optimum test species.

It is necessary to consider both quantitative and qualitative responses in laboratory animals when establishing the ADI. For example, it is recognized that compound-induced peroxisome proliferation is considerably greater in mice, rats, and hamsters than in humans [9; 176; 180]. Thus, these species may be inappropriate for investigating this effect in man. Since specific knowledge of comparative metabolism and the basis for differences in species sensitivity are often unavailable, the effects noted in the most sensitive species usually provides the basis for the ADI assessment.

JMPR, recognizing the difficulties of obtaining *in vivo* human data, has proposed as a compromise the generation of *in vitro* data using human tissues or cultured human cell lines [78]. Comparison can then be made (a) between *in vitro* data generated in a number of species and (b) between the *in vitro* and *in vivo* data in the test species. Such a procedure would markedly assist in the selection of the most appropriate species for studies involving multiple daily administrations and in the extrapolation of data. A comparison of this nature for methylene chloride has recently generated a great deal of interest and has been proposed for use in safety assessment [3].

The choice of species should also depend upon the susceptibility of the species (or strain) to the toxic effect being investigated. Thus, in teratogenic studies, the test species or strain should be known to be susceptible to teratogenic agents. As new strains of rabbits have been introduced for teratology studies, JMPR has had to request evidence (from exposure to known teratogens) of their sensitivity and hence their appropriateness for such studies, e.g., methacrifos [67]. In addition, the time of specific embryological events in different mouse strains may result in the absence of insult at crucial times in teratology studies [120].

The normal incidence of a pathological lesion may also influence the choice of test species or strain. For instance, the use of a strain in which the incidence of tumours in a particular organ is excessively high in untreated animals (e.g., the incidence of pituitary tumours in most strains of rat) would be contra-indicated if there was information indicating that elements of the endocrine system could be among the target organs (i.e., if hormonal imbalance were suspected). Similarly, the high incidence of liver tumours in control male $B6C3F_1$ mice may also mask a neoplastic response in treated animals. Thus, a thorough knowledge of the strain being considered for the study is essential to determine its suitability for a specific type of experiment.

8.2.2　Group size

Group size in toxicity studies is dependent upon a number of factors, including the purpose of the experiment, the required sensitivity of the study, the lifespan of the species under test, the design of the study, the reproductive capacity and the fertility of the species, economic aspects, and the availability of animals. This section contains a brief discussion of group sizes acceptable for various toxicity tests followed by a more detailed discussion of numbers of animals to be utilized in long term/oncogenicity studies.

In acute oral toxicity tests in rodent species, the number of animals utilized depends upon the degree of accuracy required. LD_{50} determinations (as indicated by 95% confidence limits) are approximate, rather than accurate. To obtain these approximations, five animals per sex per dose level are usually used. Because of the problems of availability and because of economic factors involved in utilizing non-rodent species, smaller numbers of non-rodents (resulting in reduced accuracy) are frequently utilized in acute toxicity studies, especially when the objective of the study is to examine the comparative toxicity between species.

In teratology studies, because the objective is to obtain adequate numbers of litters from treated females, the actual number of animals required is dependent on fertility and the difficulties encountered in breeding. Most protocols for studies with rodent species specify 20-25 pregnant females per dose level. When other species are used, such as the rabbit, smaller group sizes (usually producing a minimum of 12 litters) are utilized. However, when equivocal data are obtained from such studies (e.g., an incidence of congenital malformations, which, although not statistically significant, shows positive trend analysis), increased group size or the provision of adequate historical control data may be necessary.

In multigeneration studies in rats, a minimum of 20 pregnant females per dose level per mating are usually used. As with teratology studies, fertility and breeding ability in captivity must be considered when determining group size at each dose level. In addition, sufficient litters are required from the mating of the generation that is used as the source of parent animals for the next generation. Ideally, sufficient litters should be available at each dose level to permit selection of future parental animals for the next generation on the basis of 1 male and 1 female per litter. Again, this factor must be considered in initial determinations of group size. This ideal is not always achievable, since, if some females do not produce offspring, or a litter contains animals of only one sex, then group size will diminish as the study proceeds. Under these circumstances, the selection of parental animals for the next generation should be based on the widest distribution permissible from the available litters. It should also be noted that, if closely inbred strains are being used, the distribution of future parents becomes less critical. The limiting factor in multigeneration studies is usually the logistics of the study which, since animals do not mate or deliver to order, become increasingly complex with each mating and with each generation.

Appropriate group sizes in short-term studies depend upon the purpose of the study. These studies are often designed to provide information useful for the selection of dose levels to be used in subsequent long-term studies. They are, however, sometimes used as the basis for the ADI. In these cases, increased group size is desirable. The short-term study utilized for selection of doses in future studies requires a minimum of 10 animals of each sex per dose level in rodent species. Smaller group sizes (e.g., 4-6 of each sex per dose level) are generally accepted for non-rodent species such as the dog.

In considering long-term/oncogenicity studies, the protocol frequently separates the two components of the study. The basic group size is based on the oncogenicity study, with ancillary groups for intermediate sacrifices and for investigation of haematological, clinical chemistry, and urinalysis parameters. Group sizes must be sufficient to ensure that adequate numbers of animals survive to the termination of the study. Furthermore, the study design must be such that the sensitivity of the study, i.e., its ability to detect an adverse effect, is acceptable. A recent publication by the International Agency for Research on Cancer (IARC) [100] has addressed the sensitivity of carcinogenic studies. Tables 1 and 2, reproduced from this publication, indicate the numbers of animals of each sex per dose level required to attain specified sensitivities in a two-dose-level study. (It should be noted that three dose levels are generally required for safety assessments; see section 8.2.3).

Table 1. Minimum group sizes required to ensure a false-negative
rate of 10% or less[a]

Excess tumour incidence in test group (%)[b]	Tumour incidence in control group				
	0%	1%	5%	10%	20%
1	819	2611	9084	16 287	28 110
5	162	243	503	783	1232
10	80	100	166	233	339
15	53	61	90	119	163
20	39	44	59	75	98
25	31	34	43	53	67

[a]   Based on Fischer exact test ($p < 0.05$) with n animals in each of a control and a test group, and assuming that all animals respond independently.

[b]   Difference between the response rates in the test and the control groups, respectively.

As can be seen from these data, test sensitivity is a major factor in determining group size. Furthermore, these data emphasize the importance of the background incidence of tumours in untreated animals, which in turn underlines the importance of species or strain selection for oncogenicity studies (see section 8.2.1 and 8.2.6).

Group sizes utilized in oncogenicity studies are usually in the range of 50 to 100 animals of each sex per dose level. For additional information on group sizes in oncogenicity studies, Annex 2 of reference 176 should be consulted.

Table 2. Number of animals per group required to obtain false-positive
rates of 5% and false-negative rates of 10% based on tests for
linear trend with three equally spaced doses

Tumour response rates			Number of
Control	Low Dose	High Dose	animals/group
0.02	0.04	0.06	420
0.02	0.07	0.12	112
0.02	0.12	0.22	44
0.10	0.12	0.14	1150
0.10	0.15	0.20	224
0.10	0.20	0.30	70
0.20	0.22	0.24	1860
0.20	0.25	0.30	328
0.20	0.30	0.40	93

The size of ancillary groups depends upon the basic study protocol. The utilization of a procedure for interim kills requires sufficient animals to be sacrificed at each kill to provide adequate numbers for histological analysis. Groups designated for haematological, clinical chemistry, and urine analyses must be of adequate size for proper statistical analysis of the data that are generated and to allow for anticipated mortality as the study proceeds. In general, a minimum of 10 animals of each sex per dose level should be available for each sub-group required.

8.2.3 Selection of dose levels

Data obtained from acute toxicity studies can sometimes assist in the selection of appropriate dose levels for use in short-term feeding studies. Thus, when acute toxicity data are available, it is not unusual for some fraction of the LD_{50} or of the LD_{01} determined from acute toxicity studies to be employed. When available, data on pharmacokinetics or metabolism can be helpful in determining dose levels for short-term toxicity studies, particularly if there is evidence of bio-accumulation of the test compound or of its metabolites, or if there is evidence of dose-dependent changes in detoxification. Since the determination of a dose-response curve is one of the objectives of short-term studies, at least three dose levels are normally required, as well as a control.

The selection of dose levels in long-term or oncogenicity studies should be based on the information derived from pharmacokinetic, pharmacodynamic, and short-term toxicity studies. Frequently, the highest dose level selected is the maximum tolerated dose (MTD), estimated from short-term feeding studies. However, there are problems in attempting to extrapolate data obtained at high dose levels in experimental animals to probable human exposure levels. This concept was discussed by the 1987 JMPR, which made the following statement:

"The Meeting was concerned at (sic) the difficulties of interpretation of the results of long-term studies in which high doses had been used. In reproduction and teratology studies the use of maternally toxic doses has also caused concern. The Meeting discussed the maximum tolerated dose (MTD), which has been defined 'as a dose that does not shorten life expectancy nor produce signs of toxicity other than those due to cancer' and 'operationally, as the maximum dose level at which a substance induces a decrement in weight gain of no greater than 10% in a subchronic toxicity test' [176]. To identify agents with particularly low orders of toxicity, exposure conditions are often maximized. These may include the use of very high doses and gavage administration. A number of assumptions are implicit in the use of the MTD: (i) the absorption, distribution, biotransformation, and excretion of a chemical are not dose-dependent (that is, their kinetics are the same at low and high doses); (ii) both the rate and extent of reparative processes (for example, DNA repair) are independent of dose and of the extent of damage; (iii) the response to a chemical is not age-dependent; (iv) the dose-dependent response is linear; (v) doses tested in animals need not bear any relationship to human exposure levels." [78, p. 3].

At the 1987 JMPR meeting, these assumptions were questioned. Thus:

(i)   absorption, distribution, biotransformation, and excretion of a compound are dependent on several factors, e.g., physicochemical properties, degree of protein binding, bioavailability, and saturation of routes of metabolism (resulting in variations in the proportions of different metabolites or complete changes in metabolic pathways with dose (e.g., 2-phenylphenol));

(ii)   DNA repair is dependent on dose and/or degree of damage both in vivo and in vitro [7; 139];

(iii)   the response to many chemicals is age-dependent (e.g., acute toxicity of DDT or malathion [116]);

(iv)   the US NCTR study on 2-acetylaminofluorene (the megamouse study) did not demonstrate a linear response for bladder tumours [99];

(v)   results of studies at dose levels many orders of magnitude above the level of human exposure to pesticide residues in food have little relevance to the safety assessment of pesticide residues in the diet (e.g., 2-phenylphenol [75]).

The JMPR has indicated that, instead of using the MTD to select the top-dose level, the use of properly designed biotransformation studies over a range of doses (including human exposure levels) may provide a more rational basis for dose selection in long-term animal studies.

8.2.4   Test duration

In certain studies, e.g., teratology and multigeneration studies, the duration of the study is determined by the biological character- istics of the test species or strain. The duration of these types of studies is considered in sections 8.3.5.1 and 8.3.5.2.

The duration of other studies is determined, to some extent, by definition. Thus, an acute study was originally defined as a single- dose study, observation of the treated animal continuing for 2 to 4 weeks following dosing [37]. The concept of an acute study has changed slightly through the years; it is now considered to be a study of the effects of a dose administered either singly or on several occasions over a period of 24 hours. The observation period is usually 14 days [124].

A short-term study has been defined as having a duration lasting up to 10% of the animal's lifespan [31], 90 days in rats and mice, or 1 year in dogs. It has also been defined as a study covering less than half the animal's lifespan [37].

Long-term/oncogenicity studies are usually defined as studies last- ing for the greater part of the lifespan of the animal [176, p. 113]. Studies of this type usually fall into one of two categories: (a) a specific duration; (b) until mortality in the most susceptible group attains a fixed level, usually 80%. Fixed-term studies vary in duration with species and strain, depending on lifespan. The late development of many types of tumours requires that the study be permitted to continue as long as possible. In addition, reduced liver or kidney function with increasing age and a consequent increase in the plasma levels of toxins in older animals may result in manifestations of toxicity not otherwise seen. However, low survival rates and normal geriatric changes may complicate study interpretation and limit the sensitivity of comparison between groups. Thus, the goal of a long-term oncogenicity study is to determine the optimum balance between these factors.

The report of the 1967 WHO Scientific Group [169] concluded that it is better to terminate toxicity studies before the complications of senescence arise in the test animals. Although many effects of sen- escence are now recognized, further data are still required before scientifically supportable generalizations on the duration of long-term studies are possible. If a finite mortality is the definitive endpoint of the study, then care must be taken:

• to ensure that mortality does not exceed the predetermined limit in any group (including the control);

- to consider whether the mortality arises because of tumour development;

- that autopsies are performed as soon as possible on animals dying during the study, thereby avoiding loss of information due to autolysis or cannibalism.

8.2.5   Pathological procedures

Three steps are involved in the pathological examination of experimental animals:

- gross pathological examination at the time of post-mortem;

- histopathological examination of the tissues;

- a review of these data by an independent pathologist.

For the last of these steps, JMPR has recommended to WHO that a mechanism should be established to permit independent pathological assessment of questionable or disputed findings that are brought forward for review [65].

Pathological examinations and the way in which they are reported can give rise to a number of problems.

In acute toxicity studies, gross pathological examination of animals both dying during the study and killed at the termination of the observation period is desirable, because one of the objectives of an acute oral study is to obtain information on potential target organs and on possible dose levels to be used in subsequent repeated administration studies. Such information should, therefore, be as comprehensive as possible and should include gross pathology examination. Unfortunately, such examinations are not always performed or reported.

In short- and long-term studies, pathology is a major endpoint. However, the presentation of pathological data is often confusing. Gross pathological data (frequently reported separately from the data on histopathological examinations) are difficult to correlate with histopathological findings. It is not unusual to find gross pathological notations of "lumps and bumps", petechial haemorrhages, etc., in an organ, for which the histopathological notation is "normal". A high frequency of such apparent discrepancies in the absence of any comment is unsatisfactory. The explanation may be either a mix-up in specimens, or that the sections cut for histopathological examination failed to intersect a "lump or bump". Either way, the study probably has not achieved its objectives. Partial resolution of these problems can sometimes be achieved by cutting multiple sections throughout the area of the gross lesion.

Pathological terminology is also confusing since several different names may be used for the same lesion. Therefore, an adequate description of the lesion and an indication of its size and frequency is

essential in pathological reports. Furthermore, a standard classification of lesions should always be used in reports, e.g., the International Agency for Research on Cancer (IARC) Tumour Register [183].

A high incidence of tissue autolysis is occasionally noted in the
histopathological reports. Even fairly advanced autolysis does not
necessarily preclude the identification of a tumour, despite the fact
that the specific cellular characteristics are obscured by autolytic
activity. Although such tumours cannot always be reported in adequate
detail, their presence can be recorded.

The percentage incidence of tumours is of importance in the evaluation, but data are often such that it is extremely difficult to determine how many animals were actually examined with respect to a specific
tissue. In the absence of such information, although the number of
diagnosed tumours is known, percentage incidence cannot be determined.

The precise site of tumours may be of major importance. In a recent
evaluation of folpet, tumours in the duodenum and jejunum of the experimental animals were noted and a probable mechanism for the induction
of these tumours was proposed [77]. The data were inadequate to determine whether these tumours were a "spill-over" (related to the irri-
tant properties of the compound) or whether they were induced independently of the postulated mechanism. Additional data were required to
resolve this problem and, hence, to arrive at a valid evaluation of the
safety of the compound [76].

The increasing emphasis on mechanism of action in evaluating toxicity studies may be supported by histopathological examinations
utilizing special stains for identification of cell elements (e.g.,
Sudan III for fat droplets) or involving histochemical techniques.
Electron microscopic examination should also be considered when biochemical or other data indicate the need to examine cell organelles or
membrane structures.

Many protocols for multigeneration studies require histopathological examination of a representative selection of pups at one or more
points in the study. The need for such examination is questionable
(see section 8.3.5.1).

8.2.6   Historical control data

In almost all toxicity studies, quantitative and qualitative data
from several treated animal groups are compared with data from one or
more concurrent untreated or vehicle-treated control groups. The application of appropriate statistical procedures will indicate, with some
predetermined probability, which of the observed differences are not
likely to be attributable to chance. In such procedures, the data from
untreated animals become the standard reference. Yet it is known that,
even with random assignment of individual animals to each group and
strict adherence to GLP, the incidence of spontaneous neoplastic and
other morphologic lesions is often highly variable among control groups
of the same species and strain in different studies conducted within a

single laboratory, as well as in different laboratories [119; 152; 157; 167; 168].

To be indicative of a treatment-induced change, the differences between control and treatment groups should show a dose-response relationship and delineate a trend away from the expected norm for the particular species and strain of experimental animal used. Since data from the concurrent control group are used as the standard reference for treatment group responses, and since control data in any particular study may be unpredictably variable, qualitative and quantitative criteria must be used to evaluate whether the concurrent control data constitute the typical species/strain pattern, i.e. whether they correspond to an expected norm. Historical control data relating to the specific species/strain used in the study provides such evaluation criteria [23; 126; 154; 155]. This type of information must be viewed as an auxiliary aid to interpretation of data from the study. It should not be used as a complete substitution for concurrent control data.

The following have been proposed for use in the evaluation of carcinogenicity data by a Task Force of Past Presidents of the Society Of Toxicology [155] and may have utility for the evaluation of other forms of toxicity as well:

- If the incidence rate or other observed effect in the concurrent control group is lower than in the historical control groups but these same effects in the treated groups are within the historical control range, the differences between treated and control groups are not biologically relevant.

- If the incidence rates or other observed effects in the treated groups are higher than the historical control range but not statistically significantly greater than the concurrent control incidence, the conclusion would be that there is no relation to treatment (but with the reservation that this result could have arisen by chance or because of flaws in the assay and may therefore be a false negative).

- If the incidence rates or other observed effects in the treated groups are significantly greater than in the concurrent controls and greater than the historical control range, a treatment effect is probably present which is unlikely to be a false positive result.

The best historical control data are obtained using the same species and strain, from the same supplier, maintained under the same routine conditions in the same laboratory that generated the study data being evaluated. The data should be from control animals from contemporaneous studies. Statistical procedures can be used to relate the overall historical incidence to that in a specific study. However, this leaves much to be desired since the incidence of spontaneous lesions and the averages of quantitative data can vary considerably between groups of animals. This type of variation is not apparent if the incidence in combined historical control animals is used [157].

To assess variability, historical control data should be presented as discrete group incidences, segregated by sex and age and updated with each new study that is performed [135]. It is also highly desirable that additional information on each discrete control group be made available. This information should include the following:

- identification of species, strain, name of the supplier, and specific colony identification if the supplier has more than one geographical location;

- name of the laboratory and time during which the study was performed;

- description of general conditions under which the animals were maintained, including the type or brand of diet and, where possible, the amount consumed;

- the approximate age, in days, of the control animals at the beginning of the study and at the time of killing or death;

- description of the control group mortality pattern observed during or at the end of the study and of any other pertinent observations (e.g., diseases, infections);

- name of the pathology laboratory and the examining pathologist who was responsible for gathering and interpreting the pathological data from the study;

- what tumours may have been combined to produce any of the incidence data.

8.3 Conduct and Evaluation of Different Types of Studies

8.3.1 Short-term and long-term toxicity studies

Both short- and long-term feeding studies utilize the same methodologies and differ only in the duration of the test. The parameters investigated usually include body and organ weights, clinical chemistry and haematological effects, and gross and histopathological examinations.

Short- and long-term toxicity studies are designed to determine the NOAEL for the test substance and to provide information relevant to the determination of the safety factor to be applied in extrapolating to humans (see section 2.2).

The majority of protocols available for toxicity testing are intended as guidelines, thus leaving the final study design to the individual investigator. It is usually the case that by the time the long-term toxicity studies are initiated, the investigator will have access to the information from earlier studies (acute, short-term, and metabolic studies) and hence will be able to judge the most suitable design for long-term studies.

The selection of species and of dose levels have been discussed in sections 8.2.1 and 8.2.3.

In long-term oral toxicity studies, the test substance is normally incorporated in the diet and administered for the majority of the lifetime (see section 8.2.4), on a daily basis (7 days per week). Lifetime exposure is required due to the fact that, during the aging process, factors such as altered tissue sensitivity, changing metabolic and physiological capability, and spontaneous disease may alter the nature of the toxic response [171]. Spontaneous diseases include age-related increases in the incidence of heart disease, chronic renal failure, and neoplasia, which are observed in most mammalian species.

To ensure that the objectives of the long-term toxicity study are achieved, statistical principles must be used to determine adequate group sizes for reducing the incidence of false positives and false negatives to a minimum (section 8.2.2). Similarly, the use of random numbers or comparable statistical techniques, both for allocating animals to experimental groups and for ensuring that the distribution of cages of animals within housing racks is random, is essential to minimize bias in selecting animals and minimize possible environmental effects (e.g., temperature, humidity, light) within the animal house [176, Annex II].

In conducting these studies, the principles of GLP [161; 160] should be followed to ensure both acceptable conditions of animal husbandry and adequate conduct of the experiment. Full records on all animals must be kept, detailing all observations, results of any laboratory techniques (e.g., bleeding and subsequent haematological or clinical chemistry studies), and information on pathological examinations at the end of the study.

Since one of the objectives of a feeding study is to determine changes in toxic signs and manifestations, it is axiomatic that periodic detailed examinations be performed on at least a proportion of the experimental animals. Non-invasive procedures such as the measurement of body weight and food consumption, palpation, behavioural observations, and assessment of general condition of the experimental animals (both control and exposed) can be performed regularly. The frequency of handling may be limited by the potential for creating stress in the experimental animal, particularly if the frequency is increased towards termination of the study (i.e. in oncogenicity studies). Urinalysis, the remaining routine non-invasive technique, should also be performed regularly, but at longer time intervals (usually at 3, 6, 12, 18, and 24 months in rat studies). The process of collecting urine may cause stress, depending upon the type of caging used. Thus, if animals are housed one per cage, the use of metabolism cages for single animals will induce minimal stress. However, where multiple caging is the norm, sudden isolation can induce a stress condition, with consequent physiological changes in the animal. This should be considered when the results of urinalysis are interpreted.

In general, urinalysis utilizes insufficient animals (often as few as five of each sex per dose level) or an insufficient acclimatization period in the metabolism cage(s) to be very useful, since variability, even in the same individual, can be high [150]. Even if the numbers of animals or acclimatization time is adequate, further problems may be encountered. Dissolved carbon dioxide may dissipate and thus alter pH, the appearance of the urine may vary according to the time of day at which sampling takes place, and bacterial concentration and composition may change even if preservatives are used. However, useful data can be obtained in clinical chemistry studies on urine, such as concentrations of proteins, ketones (elevated in starvation or with low carbohydrate diets), glucose (diabetes, hypoglycaemia), and porphyrins (elevated with liver disorders), osmolality (reflecting kidney function, but data on water consumption is needed to interpret kidney concentration effects), urinary haemoglobin (often elevated in toxic situations), and high crystal content (possibly predictive of kidney or bladder stones). In addition, periodic urine collection and analysis for metabolites of the test substance may yield data on age-related changes in metabolism.

Invasive techniques (usually involving blood sampling) normally utilize a pre-designated ancillary group of animals identified for that purpose prior to the onset of the study. Thus the effects of repeated bleeding at specific intervals (the intervals usually being similar to those delineated for urinalysis) on terminal pathological manifestations are recognizable in animals in the ancillary group. The ancillary groups (which must allow for mortality with increasing duration of the study) should comprise at least 12 animals of each sex per dose level for each group to provide groups of at least 10 animals of each sex per dose level for haematological and other clinical chemistry examinations.

End-points normally measured in haematological examinations include erythrocyte counts, leucocyte counts, differential leucocyte counts, haemoglobin, haematocrit, and platelet and reticulocyte counts. In addition, erythrocyte fragility, sedimentation rate, and coagulation factors are frequently measured and bone marrow is examined.

End-points traditionally examined by clinical chemistry measurements include:

• serum bilirubin (liver and haematological effects);

• serum glucose;

• lactate dehydrogenase (a non-specific indicator of tissue damage seen in myocardial infarction, renal toxicity, pulmonary embolism, and pernicious anaemia);

• serum alkaline phosphatase (which, it should be noted, decreases with age and with nutritional status, and cannot be regarded as specifically indicative of a disease process because of its wide distribution in many organs);

- alanine aminotransferase (previously serum glutamic-pyruvic transaminase) and aspartate aminotransferase (previously serum glutamic-oxalic transaminase) (both indicators of liver toxicity);

- amylase (increased in renal insufficiency and pancreatitis, decreased with hepatobiliary toxicity);

- creatinine (renal failure);

- creatinine phosphorylase (elevated with myocardial infarction and lung disorders);

- cholinesterase (decreased by organophosphates and carbamates);

- serum protein;

- blood urea nitrogen (elevated with renal toxicity, depressed with liver toxicity);

- serum electrolytes (see reference [93] for a comprehensive discussion of the interpretation of clinical chemistry measurements).

It has been proposed that clinical chemistry studies be aimed mainly at known target organs that are identified in short-term toxicity studies [150]. However, long-term toxicity studies may result in changes in the degree of toxicity to specific organs (e.g., adaptation of initial target organs, secondary effects arising from the initial effects noted in short-term studies, and changes in circulating enzyme or hormone levels due to tumour development). Consequently, limiting clinical chemistry studies to parameters suggested by short-term studies is not encouraged.

In certain cases, clinical chemistry studies may be necessary to investigate endocrine organ function. For example, delayed growth or metabolic dysfunction may be the result of thyroid dysfunction, induced either by direct toxic action of the test material on the thyroid or by decreased thyrotropin release by the pituitary. Similarly, altered liver carbohydrate metabolism may be due to pancreatic dysfunction, adrenal dysfunction may result in disturbed kidney function, changes in fertility or reproductive performance may be mediated by gonadal hormonal changes, and tumour formation may arise due to enhanced hormonal stimulation, either in endocrine organs or in non-endocrine organs (e.g., the mammary gland). A recent publication [163] discusses the practical problems and describes methods of investigating endocrine toxicity.

While clinical chemistry data are often non-specific, they do permit the progress of an effect to be followed *in vivo*. When histopathological data are available (usually only at the times of interim and terminal sacrifices), they may supersede clinical chemistry findings.

The pathological data derived from feeding studies are of paramount importance. Such data in long-term feeding studies should be obtained from at least two specified sacrifice periods, one (usually a minimum of 10 rats of each sex per dose) at a point in time prior to the onset of senescence and the second at termination of the study. All animals (including all non-scheduled deaths, or animals sacrificed in a moribund condition) should be examined at least grossly, and tissues should be preserved where possible for histological examination. To avoid undue loss of tissues due to autolysis, animals should be checked at least 2 or 3 times daily. A high incidence of autolyzed animals results in loss of data and raises concerns about the quality of the animal husbandry and standard of laboratory expertise.

Histopathological examination should cover a wide range of organs and tissues. However, recognizing the economics of histopathological examinations, examination of tissues from mid- and low-dose groups may be limited to those tissues where differences occurred between those from control and high-dose groups.

The NOAEL is frequently based on the results of the pathological examination of the test animals. The initial (gross) examination notes any abnormalities in the tissues (e.g., masses, discoloration, necrosis). This is followed by removal and weighing of specific organs. Because of the high rate of autolysis of some organs (e.g., the kidney), removal, weighing, and preservation should be performed as rapidly as is consistent with accurate work. Paired organs should be weighed separately to avoid inaccuracies arising from unilateral lesions (e.g., tumours) that are not grossly visible. Organs normally weighed include the liver, kidneys, heart, adrenals, gonads, spleen, and brain. Results of such weighings should be reported as absolute weights, and also as a ratio to body weight and to brain weight.

In assessing data from short- and long-term toxicity studies, the following factors should be considered:

- Comparison of mean values of body weights for specific groups of animals may not necessarily be the most appropriate method of detecting potentially toxic effects. The use of body weight gain differences should also be considered, as should changes in food intake.

- Clinical chemistry data can provide a useful indicator of toxicological effects. However, they are limited in sensitivity and frank pathological changes are often observed at dose levels less than or equal to those resulting in significant clinical chemistry effects. When studies include a post-treatment recovery period, clinical chemistry data are frequently of value in assessing the progress of recovery. In many cases, the specificity of the test system, e.g., serum alkaline phosphatase, is insufficient to permit precise identification of target tissues or organs. In other cases, e.g., acetylcholinesterase measurements, clinical chemistry data may be the major toxicological effect measured.

• Changes in a single haematological parameter unsupported by further changes in other haematological parameters or by pathological changes in bone marrow or spleen are rarely of toxicological significance.

• Organ weight changes should always be examined on an absolute and organ/body weight ratio basis. Organ/body weight ratios can be misleading when a change in body weight occurs. Mathematical procedures for correcting for this situation exist. When the body weight *per se* is affected, there is a tendency to place greater reliance on organ/brain weight ratios.

• Gross and histopathological examinations should be carefully checked for correspondence. A detailed description of the lesion(s) or photomicrographs may be necessary since the terminology used for certain lesions is variable and there is some degree of subjectivity in the interpretation of lesions (see also section 8.2.5).

No discussion of toxicity studies would be complete without some consideration of the dose actually ingested. Dose-level selection is discussed in section 8.2.3 and stability of the test material in the diet in section 4. Assuming that the stability is acceptable and that the homogeneity of the test material in the diet has been measured on a number of occasions during the study, one major variable remains, i.e. the food consumption per unit of body weight. This varies with age, being highest in the young animal and decreasing as the animal ages (the special case of lactating females is discussed in section 8.3.3.1). When data are available, the actual dose ingested is calculated from the concentration of test substance in the diet and the food consumption. Under these circumstances, the JMPR evaluation indicates the NOAEL as X ppm *equal* to Y mg/kg body weight per day, and is usually based on the mean intake of the test substance over the lifespan. In other cases, when the calculation of intake in mg/kg body weight per day is not feasible because of inadequate food intake data, the JMPR evaluation uses the standard conversion factors for ppm to mg/kg body weight per day ([114], reproduced as Annex II in this monograph), this being reported as X ppm *equivalent* to Y mg/kg body weight per day. The former method is preferable.

8.3.2   Carcinogenicity studies

From its inception, JMPR has recognized the need to evaluate the carcinogenicity of pesticide residues in food [32]. It has adopted the principle that carcinogenicity testing should utilize adequate numbers of animals, generally of two or more species (e.g., rat and mouse), and a suitably high dose level of the substance should be fed for the lifetime of the animals [33].

8.3.2.1   Background

The 1977 Joint Meeting noted that an evaluation of carcinogenicity should be undertaken routinely for:

- pesticides whose use results in substantial residues in crops directly or indirectly used for human food;

- pesticides with structural similarity to known carcinogens;

- pesticides that are metabolized to, or leave residues that are, known carcinogens or closely related to such compounds;

- pesticides that give rise to early pathology suggestive of potential tumorigenicity;

- pesticides with pharmacokinetic properties "suggestive of covalent binding to tissues" or bioaccumulation [57].

JMPR has sometimes recommended that certain compounds should not be used where residues may occur in food, due to their potential carcinogenicity (e.g., hexachlorobenzene, captafol). At other times, either TADIs or ADIs have been set, even though there was limited evidence of carcinogenicity in animals (e.g., several chlorinated organic insecticides). Overall, JMPR has maintained the philosophy that a pesticide for which there is limited evidence of carcinogenicity should not necessarily be prohibited (see section 8.3.2.7).

8.3.2.2   Routes of exposure

The oral route of administration is the most appropriate one for determining in experimental animals the carcinogenic potential of pesticides leaving residues in food.

The 1966 JMPR [38] noted the comments of the report of a WHO Scientific Group [169] concerning experimentally induced local sarcomas that apparently result from the physical characteristics of the test material. This Joint Meeting concluded that for the routine testing of pesticide residues, the subcutaneous route is not generally appropriate. The occurrence of local sarcomas following subcutaneous injection should not alone be considered sufficient evidence of a carcinogenic hazard following ingestion [169]. It does, however, indicate that further studies would be desirable.

The 1989 JMPR noted that severe local effects may interfere with the interpretation of data, e.g., the production of forestomach epithelial hyperplasia and papilloma formation following the administration of gastric irritants. It was recommended that methods of administration other than feeding be justified.

*8.3.2.3   Commonly   occurring   tumours   and   factors   influencing   tumour
incidence in different species*

Some rodents commonly used for *in vivo* bioassays exhibit high incidences of some tumours. In evaluating toxicological data, it is important to determine whether an increased incidence of tumours and/or a
decreased time to tumour in exposed animals are related to treatment.
The incidence of such tumours in control animals may vary considerably
with time. As an example, ten years ago the occurrence of Leydig cell
tumours in rats was rarely reported. By 1987, some laboratories were
reporting that the occurrence of such tumours sometimes reached 50% in
control rats. It is not known whether this change in incidence is due
to a genetic shift in certain rat strains or to more careful pathological examinations of the rat testes. The importance of such factors is
discussed in section 8.2.6.

As noted in Environmental Health Criteria 70 [176]:

"The evaluation of studies in which commonly-occurring tumours are
a complicating factor needs careful individual assessment. The tumours
that have given rise to the most controversy in recent years are hepatomas (particularly in the mouse), pheochromocytomas in the rat (see
below), lymphomas and lung adenomas in the mouse, pancreatic adenomas
and gastric papillomas in the rat, and certain endocrine-associated
tumours, including pituitary, mammary, and thyroid tumours in both rats
and mice. Some of these tumours, such as hepatomas and lung adenomas,
may occur in the majority of untreated animals.

"With the exception of lymphomas, some of which are virally
associated, the endocrine-associated tumours, and possibly hepatomas in
high-incidence strains of mice, which may involve oncogenes [82], there
is no clue as to the origin of tumours that occur commonly in exper-
imentally-used rodents. Indeed, there is not even any cogent specu-
lation as to the mechanisms by which these tumour incidences are
increased." [176, p. 44].

Since the publication of Environmental Health Criteria 70, a great
deal of additional research has been carried out on the etiology of
cancer, particularly with respect to the important role of oncogenes in
neoplasia. Nevertheless, additional investigation into the initiation,
promotion, and progression of cancer is necessary to assist the incor-
poration of such mechanistic considerations into human hazard assessment for carcinogens.

JMPR has generally considered it unwise to classify a compound as a
carcinogen solely on the basis of an increased incidence of tumours of
a kind that commonly occur spontaneously in the species and strain
under study and at a frequency that may seriously reduce the statistical power of the study. Data are usually required in one or preferably
two alternate species, and the overall evidence is then considered.

The significance of mouse liver tumours was first considered by the
1970 JMPR [46]. These tumours were then becoming more frequently

observed in carcinogenicity studies, especially following exposure to the chlorinated organic pesticides. Subsequent Joint Meetings [46; 48; 52; 53; 57; 72; 74] have also considered the problem of pesticides that induce mouse hepatic tumours. A number of hypotheses concerning the etiology of mouse liver tumours have been considered by JMPR [2; 132; 133; 162; 170]. Biochemical differences between the mouse and many other species, including humans, are highly pertinent to mouse hepatomas [72]. In addition, degranulation of endoplasmic reticulum is known to be associated with carcinogenesis in the mouse [130; 131; 134]. Both dieldrin and phenobarbitone degranulate the hepatic endoplasmic reticulum of CF1 mice, a strain susceptible to dieldrin-induced tumorigenesis, but do not degranulate the endoplasmic reticulum of LACG mice, a non-susceptible strain, nor that of rats or humans. The current position of JMPR is that mouse liver tumours are of little relevance in predicting human cancer risk. It is inadvisable to classify a substance as likely to be a carcinogen to humans solely on the basis of an increased incidence of mouse liver tumours [72].

Other tumours occurring with a high relative frequency are adrenal medullary lesions in rats. As noted in Environmental Health Criteria 70 [176]:

"An overview of the literature indicates that untreated rats of various strains may exhibit widely differing incidences of lesions described as 'pheochromocytomas' [69; 141; 142]. There are no clear criteria for distinguishing between prominent foci of hyperplasia and benign neoplasms, and pathologists differ in the criteria that they use for distinguishing between benign and malignant adrenal medullary tumours.

"Rats fed *ad libitum* on highly nutritious diets tend to develop a wide variety of neoplasms, particularly of the endocrine glands, in much higher incidences than animals provided with enough food to meet their nutritional needs but not enough to render them obese. The adrenal medulla is just one of the sites affected by overfeeding. Controlled feeding . . . reduces the life-time expectation of developing either hyperplasia or neoplasia of the adrenal medulla in rats." [176, p. 44].

Thus, food intake can be a major factor in experimental carcinogenesis. Restricted food intake in rodents is known to increase life expectancy and to reduce the incidence of naturally occurring and some induced tumours. However, restricted dietary intake may also require other considerations (e.g., study duration) be taken into account in designing protocols for carcinogenicity studies.

8.3.2.4 *Pathological classification of neoplasms*

The need for guidelines leading to consistency in pathological diagnosis is apparent. As noted in Environmental Health Criteria 70 [176], tumours should be classified and analyzed on the basis of their histogenic origin in order to prevent different malignant tumours, occurring in the same organ, from being grouped inappropriately for statistical analysis. This is particularly important when brain tumour incidences are being considered, since different tumour types are frequently, but incorrectly, grouped together for analysis.

Accurate determination of histogenic origin is clearly important in determining the significance of benign tumours, since this is often a complicating factor in assessing carcinogenicity studies. As noted in Environmental Health Criteria 70:

"If benign and malignant tumours are observed in an animal tissue and there is evidence of progression from the benign to the malignant state, then it is appropriate to combine the tumour types before performing statistical analysis. It is, however, still advisable to examine incidences of benign and malignant tumours separately. Assessment of the relative numbers of benign and malignant tumours at the various dose levels in the study can help determine the dose response of the animal to the compound under test. On the other hand, if only benign tumours are observed and there is no indication that they progress to malignancy, then, in most cases, it is not appropriate to consider the compound to be a frank carcinogen, under the conditions of the test (this finding may suggest further study)." [176, pp. 44-45].

The 1983 JMPR [70] indicated possible approaches (e.g., interim sacrifice of satellite groups, morphometric measurement of tumours) to the problem of latency, which is an important component of the evaluation of carcinogenic potential.

8.3.2.5 Evaluation of carcinogenicity studies

Various classification schemes have been proposed for potential chemical carcinogens. For example, IARC Working Groups evaluate evidence on the carcinogenicity of agents in humans and describe them in standard terms of "sufficient", "limited", or "inadequate" evidence of carcinogenicity or "evidence suggesting lack of carcinogenicity". These categories refer only to the strength of the evidence that an agent is carcinogenic and not to the extent of its carcinogenic activity (potency) nor to the mechanisms involved. Finally the total body of evidence (including, where relevant, supporting evidence of carcinogenicity from other data such as genetic and related effects) from humans and experimental systems is taken into account and an agent is categorized into one of four groups [101]:

Group 1: carcinogenic to humans,

Group 2A: probably carcinogenic to humans,

Group 2B: possibly carcinogenic to humans,

Group 3: not classifiable as to carcinogenicity to humans, and

Group 4: probably not carcinogenic to humans.

JMPR considers, where possible, both carcinogenic potency and biological relevance in its evaluations. It does not utilize a classification system for carcinogenic pesticides, preferring to evaluate compounds on a case-by-case basis, rather than allocating a compound to "the best fit" position in existing classification systems.

8.3.2.6   *Extrapolation from animals to man*

Different approaches to the extrapolation of animal carcinogenicity data to humans have been utilized. One of these approaches relies on a knowledge of the comparative metabolism in the test species and in humans. If data are available indicating that a crucial metabolic pathway is overloaded, an increase in tumour incidence occurring only at dose levels exceeding those resulting in the overload, then confidence in the NOAEL is increased. If comparative metabolic data indicate a similar situation in humans, the task of extrapolation is simplified.

Another approach is based on pathological considerations. When data are available to demonstrate a fixed pattern of tumour development (e.g., progression from hyperplasia, through nodular hyperplasia and benign tumour, to malignant tumour), then a dose level below that resulting in the initial pathological change is unlikely to be carcinogenic (see also section 13.5).

In 1969, JMPR [44] urged the consideration of dose-response relationships and possible NOAELs for carcinogens. The 1974 JMPR [53] adopted several of the principles put forth by a WHO Scientific Group [170] concerning preliminary changes such as hyperplasia, the effects of hormonal compounds, and tumours apparently induced by the physical character of the carcinogen. The 1974 Joint Meeting noted that preliminary changes such as hyperplasia are associated with a number of carcinogenic compounds. Furthermore, some chemicals apparently give rise to neoplasms only after the induction of a particular pathological effect [19].

The 1983 JMPR recognized that most of the mechanisms of chemical carcinogenesis were not fully understood. In view of the uncertainty surrounding the use of various mathematical models for carcinogenicity assessment, the Meeting decided that the use of safety factors remained a reasonable approach. It also recognized the importance of taking into account all biological activities of such agents in arriving at a safety assessment. This pragmatic approach is used by JMPR in the absence of satisfactory alternatives (see section 9.2).

In determining the acceptable level of pesticide residues for humans, the safety factor utilized reflects the confidence in the data base and the degree of concern for the toxic effect. This is especially true for carcinogenic effects. Where there is the need for a very high safety factor due to concern about the safety of the pesticide, it may be prudent to recommend that the pesticide should not be used where residues in food may occur.

8.3.2.7   Principles

1. An evaluation of carcinogenicity should be undertaken for those pesticides that:

    •   may give rise to substantial residues in crops used directly or indirectly for human food;

    •   have a chemical structure similar to known carcinogens or give rise to metabolites or residues that are known carcinogens or closely related compounds;

    •   give rise to histological changes that are suggestive of potential neoplasia.

2. The oral route of administration to experimental animals is the most appropriate route for determining the carcinogenicity of pesticide residues in food.

3. All available data should be considered in the evaluation and assessment of carcinogenic activity.

4. A pesticide for which there is limited evidence of carcinogenicity in animals should not necessarily be prohibited for use.

5. Mechanistic considerations are of major importance in the extrapolation of animal carcinogenicity data to humans.

8.3.3   Reproduction studies

Multigeneration reproduction studies and teratology studies are routinely required for pesticides. Although experimental designs exist that combine teratology studies with reproduction studies, these two types of study will be considered separately in this monograph.

8.3.3.1   Multigeneration reproduction studies

The 1961 FAO/WHO Meeting on Consumer Safety in Relation to Pesticide Residues stated that one of the aims of toxicological investigations of a pesticide is to ascertain "the amount of pesticide to which man and farm animals can be exposed daily for a lifetime" [32, p. 10]. With respect to the effect of age on toxicity, a WHO Scientific Group stated: "In general, but not invariably, the young animal is more sensitive to the toxic effects of exposure to chemicals" [169, p. 10]. It also pointed out the effects of different gut flora and changes in enzymes with age (e.g., poorly developed mixed-function oxidase enzymes in newborn rodents). The Group indicated that "pertinent information observed from reproductive (multigeneration) studies provides some assurance on the safety of compounds which might be present in the diet of babies" [169, p. 12] and concluded that "useful information may be obtained from studies in newborn or young animals, from reproduction studies and biochemical studies" [169, p. 23]. It also indicated the need for further studies on "the development of enzyme systems in the human young, with particular emphasis on those enzymes responsible for dealing with foreign chemicals" [169, p. 25].

JMPR addressed the problem of toxicity to juveniles indirectly in 1963 when it stated in its report that "the Meeting considered that foods, such as milk, which figure largely in the diets of babies and invalids, should be essentially free from pesticide residues" [35, p. 6]. However, it was not until 1976 that JMPR indicated that reproduction studies should be available as part of the basic toxicology data package required for allocating an ADI [55]. The need for such studies was repeated in subsequent Meetings [59; 60; 62; 65; 67; 70; 72; 74]. It should be noted, however, that multigeneration studies on a number of compounds had been submitted and evaluated before that time, some as early as 1963 (e.g., aldrin, dieldrin, heptachlor epoxide).

In evaluating a multigeneration study, there is a tendency to focus on the conceptus, the neonate, and the immature animal, because of the known variations in toxicity in these stages of development compared to those observed in adult animals. It must also be recognized that profound physical, physiological, and psychological changes occur during pregnancy, which may affect the susceptibility of the dam to the toxicity of a specific chemical. Attention must therefore be given to maternal toxicity during pregnancy and lactation.

A number of basic protocols for the conduct of multigeneration studies have been developed [92; 125; 159; 162; 174]. None, however, have gained unanimous approval and proposals for alternatives continue to be suggested [16; 112; 128; 129].

The multigeneration study may best be viewed as a screening test for toxicity in reproducing animals because, although the emphasis is on detecting effects specific to reproduction, it is also useful for detecting the enhancement of general toxic effects that may occur as a consequence of physiological changes associated with reproduction and development.

The major asset of a multigeneration study that is well designed, conducted, and interpreted is that it has the ability to detect a wide range of indirect or direct effects on reproduction. This ability arises from the complex integration of reproductive processes, so that minimal effects that may be difficult to demonstrate in isolation may combine and cascade to generate a more notable deviation in a more distal end-point (e.g., litter weight). Observations in the premating period provide a setting for assessing subsequent observations; initial observations during mating can identify lack of libido or a disturbance of hormone (oestrous) cycles. Subsequent data are generated to indicate effects on fertility, fecundity, prenatal toxicity, parturition, lactation, weaning, and postnatal growth and development of offspring through puberty to maturity. However, those features that enhance the ability of the study to detect an effect have the disadvantage of making it difficult to ascertain the primary cause when an effect is obtained. Where multigeneration studies provide an indication of an effect on reproduction, it is usually advisable, or even mandatory, to perform follow-up studies for further elucidation. Recent proposals [112; 128; 129] seek to alleviate this limitation of protocols currently in use by allowing flexibility of operation once an effect has been detected or is suspected. A wide range of options is available for follow-up studies, including separate male and female studies, use of the three segment designs applied in drug testing, and use of the dominant lethal assay as a male fertility study.

A number of factors in the experimental design of multigeneration studies have been, or are, points of controversy. The following examples may be cited:

(a) The duration of the pre-treatment period of the first generation (F_0) has been the subject of much discussion. A period equal to one spermatic cycle plus epididymal transit time is generally used for males and a period of five estrous cycles is advised for females. A period of 100 days prior to pairing was originally proposed. However, in some rat strains, such a prolonged treatment period results in the test animals having passed peak reproductive capacity by the time mating is initiated. At present, a 70-day pre-mating treatment period is generally used. If two breeding generations are employed, the problem becomes largely academic, since the second (F_1) generation cannot reproduce until it reaches maturity and it will have been exposed continuously throughout development to sexual maturity.

(b) The need for second litters in each generation has also been a subject of controversy. Two recent studies [20; 113] indicate that second litters are more sensitive, with respect to certain parameters, than are first litters. However, although the sensitivity of the second litters is increased in some areas, there are no recorded cases where effects been observed that were not present in the first litters. Thus, provided adequate dose levels are utilized and no adverse effects are recorded in the first litter, a second litter should not be necessary. Exceptions to this generalization apply to studies in which findings in the first litter are equivocal. They also apply when compounds with long biological half-lives are being tested and plateau levels have not been attained at the time of first mating.

(c) Litter size in multigeneration studies is often "standardized" (i.e. culled, usually to eight pups on day 4 post partum). Culling may introduce bias and reduce sensitivity. Surveys of routine studies show that some supposed advantages of culling (e.g., prevention of high mortality in large litters and reduced variability of pup weight) are more imagined than real. If first litters are culled and it is suspected that this may have masked the detection of an effect, then production of a second unculled litter in the same generation is recommended.

(d) The requirement for histopathological examination of pups at weaning has also been a point of discussion. The majority of histo-pathological changes will normally be similar to those seen in routine short- or long-term studies. The need for histological examination should be on a case-by-case basis, depending upon the results of the other available studies and gross observations.

(e) It has been proposed that, since the food intake in the female rat during lactation may be as much as 2.5-fold higher than in the non-lactating female rat, it would be reasonable to reduce the level of test substance in the diet during this period, in order to give a more constant exposure in terms of mg/kg body weight. However, this is not considered advisable as a routine procedure because the study would no longer model the human situation, in which maternal exposure to pesticide residues increases during lactation. Such a procedure adds complexity to the study and complicates extrapolation of the results to humans.

The evaluation of the data from the multigeneration study starts with a scan of the entire study for effects and then focuses in more detail on specific areas, bearing in mind the following points:

(a) Data from the premating period (and from other toxicity studies) provide the baseline information against which effects on reproduction *per se* are compared. These data provide a check on whether the exposures were too high or too low or whether the interval between dosages were too wide to establish dose-related responses of any effect. The better the baseline information, the more reliable the judgements on subsequent reproductive effects.

(b) Data from the initiation of mating to parturition provide, with respect to adults, information on libido, precoital time, fertility, fecundity, duration of gestation, parturition and toxicity to the pregnant female. With respect to the offspring, litter values (size, number of live pups, and pup weight) at birth provide information that would indicate prenatal toxicity.

(c) Data from birth to weaning provide information on the potential susceptibility of the lactating female to the test substance and its effect on her nursing ability. Pup weight and survival allow the assessment of effects on postnatal growth, toxins transmitted via the milk, and development of the offspring. Effects seen during this period could be delayed responses to earlier (prenatal) insult or a combination of post- and pre-natal effects.

(d) Data on the offspring during the period from weaning to puberty provide information on the persistence or permanence of earlier effects and on direct effects on the still-immature animal. The profound changes associated with puberty provide a stress point for the detection of delayed manifestation of earlier, latent effects or enhancement of direct effects.

Comparison of results obtained from the two parental generations may be informative. The F_0 parental animals (first parental generation) have not been exposed to the test material *in utero* during lactation or during early post-weaning development, whereas the F_1 parents (second parental generation), have been exposed throughout development. Consequently, if an effect is observed (on fertility, libido, parental body weight, or general condition), comparison between the F_0 and F_1 parental animal data may yield useful information on the time at which the effect is initiated. Thus, because oocyte development is completed in the female prior to birth, adverse effects on fertility observed only in female F_1 parents would suggest that an area for further investigation would be the *in utero* oogenesis. Similarly, disturbance in the development of male hormonal systems *in utero* may be produced (e.g., fenarimol [99]), resulting in reduced libido of the F_1 males.

In considering fertility, the protocol chosen often has a marked influence on the ability to determine which sex is involved. Protocols vary with regard to methods of pairing (e.g., one male to one female, one male to two females), duration of pairing (1-3 oestrus cycles), use of replacement males in non-successful pairings, follow-up of apparently infertile males, and use of proven males. Cross-matings of untreated males with treated females and *vice versa* may be required to ascertain the sex of the infertile partner. Once this is determined, histopathological examination of the reproductive organs may yield information indicating the type of effect. Studies may also be performed on circulating hormone levels. Further details on these types of studies are given in reference [166].

The initial data on newborn pups are usually limited to the number of pups born alive. Data on stillbirths and the number of malformed pups may be inaccurate because of cannibalism. Thus, although a multigeneration study may give indications of high prenatal losses and developmental toxicity, it cannot be considered to be a definitive teratology study. Often the only indicator of prenatal developmental toxicity in the reproduction study is reduced litter size at the time of the first observation, usually several hours after parturition. However, if dose levels administered in the multigeneration study are sufficiently high, then the lack of any effect provides some reassurance regarding potential teratogenicity. Furthermore, the continuous exposure to the test substance over a long period of time in the multigeneration feeding study may lead to changes in metabolism. It may also lead to changes in the dose of parent compound or metabolite reaching the placenta or fetus or to higher blood plasma levels in the case of chemicals with long half-lives. This can lead to divergence, in either direction, of the results of multigeneration and prenatal toxicity (teratogenicity) studies.

The rate of growth and survival of post-partum pups may be affected by a number of factors including general maternal care, effects initiated *in utero*, reduced lactation by the mother, or the presence of toxicants in the milk. When the need to determine the cause of pup mortality or reduced pup weight gain arises, the initial step is usually histopathological examination of pups failing to survive. If lactation has been affected (either in terms of quantity or quality of the milk), the normal routine for investigation is cross-fostering of pups, in which pups from treated mothers are weaned by untreated maternal animals and *vice versa*.

It needs to be borne in mind that the sensitivity of the reproduction study is low for specific end-points. This is particularly true for discrete end-points such as infertility and total litter loss. Where such end-points are concerned, more sensitive indicators must be found or the dimensions of the study must be greatly increased. For example, if male infertility is suspected, studies of sperm motility, mobility, and morphology may be undertaken. In the case of male-mediated reproductive toxicity, the commonly used multigeneration study design is particularly insensitive and specialized studies are necessary if male fertility is believed to be effected. Sperm measurements are now being conducted in conjunction with some short- and long-term studies and this may partially alleviate this problem.

In addition, a commonly available, and sometimes neglected, source of supporting information may be provided by histopathological examination of the reproductive organs (after proper fixation) in the chronic toxicity studies.

8.3.3.2 Teratology studies

In 1967, the WHO Scientific Group on Procedures for Investigating Intentional and Unintentional Food Additives [169] stated that "at present, no specific tests can be recommended for the detection of teratogens, but some safeguard can be provided by multigeneration studies" [169, p. 24]. In 1976 [57] and more recently [59; 60; 62; 64; 65; 67; 70; 72; 74], JMPR has stated that teratology studies should be an integral part of the toxicology data base required for evaluation and for allocation of the ADI.

The basic teratology study (also defined by IPCS as an embryo/feto-toxicity study) involves the treatment of the pregnant animal throughout the period of organogenesis. Since this begins at or around implantation of the blastocyst into the endometrium, pre-implantation losses are not usually of concern. However, an "apparent" pre-implantation loss could be a failure to detect blastocyst implantation losses.

The route of exposure, in teratology as in other studies, can markedly influence results. The most frequent routes of administration for pesticides are diet, drinking water, or gavage. The latter, however, may result in marked differences in kinetics following the bolus administration of a high dose relative to more frequent intakes of small amounts. Thus benomyl is teratogenic when administered by gavage but not when administered via the diet [70]. This is believed to be due to the short-term high plasma levels resulting from gavage administration, compared to the much lower sustained levels which result from dietary administration. Effects following gavage administration are not always more severe than those resulting from dietary inclusion. For example, thalidomide administered to rats by gavage provides essentially negative results whereas administration in the diet in a reproduction study induces almost complete embryolethality. Comparative pharmacokinetic studies are useful and often essential for relating the findings in teratology studies to human dietary exposure.

The species most commonly used in teratology studies are the rat, the mouse, and the rabbit. More than one species is generally utilized in attempting to assess teratogenic potential because of the variability in species sensitivity. Species differences arise because of variations in metabolism, types of placentation, and in the rates and patterns of fetal development. As with other toxicity studies, more weight should be given to results in species that give the closest approximation to humans in terms of kinetics, dynamics, and other relevant parameters.

The choice of dose levels in teratology studies has recently become a point of major concern. In several publications [108; 109; 110], it has been stated that maternal toxicity is associated with species-specific patterns of malformations. These associations have often led to false presumptions of cause and effect and, further, to the presumption or implication that embryonic effects associated with maternal toxicity are unimportant. However, in such associations it is more probable that effects on the embryo and dam are independent or mutually interactive. In practical terms the conceptus and dam are indivisible and are best considered as a unit. A presumed and even proven cause and effect relationship provides only an explanation of the mechanism of action, it does not necessarily preclude the risk. For example, effects induced by alcohol, lead, or methylmercury show that, even though these effects occur at doses that induce maternal toxicity, they remain of relevance for making decisions regarding safety. In considering the choice of the highest dose level in teratology studies, it is important to note that: (a) maternal toxicity can and does occur without inducing malformations, and (b) malformations can occur without maternal toxicity being induced. Thus, at the present state of knowledge, it may be prudent to continue to utilize high dose levels which induce minimal maternal toxicity. Further research regarding the role of maternal stress in the induction of developmental toxicity is recommended.

In interpreting the significance of malformations and other structural variants, it is important to consider the stage of development of the fetus at examination. Under routine experimental conditions, the offspring are removed from the mother 12 to 24 hours before anticipated parturition to avoid the possibility of cannibalization. However, the accuracy of estimating the age of the offspring at the time of removal is questionable, since vaginal smears are normally taken only once per day, thereby reducing the accuracy of the estimation of the onset of pregnancy. Furthermore, delays in the rate of development may occur. For most malformations this is relatively unimportant. The incidence of minor variants (e.g., ossification variants) may, however, be markedly altered, especially if the compound affects the rate of development.

Dose-related minor changes should not be ignored, since they are of considerable value in assessing whether a low incidence of malformation is compound-related or coincidental. The association between changes in the pattern of minor anomalies and malformations has been amply illustrated in the past. However, considerable variability exists among laboratories in both the reporting and the assessment of these minor structural deficiencies, which renders interpretation of some studies extremely difficult. A consistently higher standard of reporting of minor anomalies is encouraged. Minor anomalies are not necessarily of great concern, however, in the absence of other manifestations of developmental toxicity.

Hydroureter and hydronephrosis are frequently associated with delayed opening of the ureter at the point of entry into the bladder, with a subsequent hydrostatic effect. Even when the incidence of these conditions is high in pre-partum fetuses, they may not be apparent in 4-day-old post-partum pups [179]. Further research is encouraged in the development of protocols for the postnatal assessment of developmental toxicity.

8.3.3.3   Screening studies in teratology

Studies in which non-mammalian species or mammalian organs and tissue cultures are used to attempt to predict teratogenicity in mammalian systems are not generally of value in safety assessments at present. Although some tests may be useful as preliminary screens to prioritize compounds for further investigation, none of the available techniques can be considered definitive studies. These techniques, however, are of value in follow-up studies to determine the mechanism of action of compounds demonstrating positive effects in standard *in vivo* studies, or as support studies.

Further discussion of screening teratology studies will be found in references [91] and [174].

8.3.3.4   Principles

1. Tests in reproducing animals are essential for the complete safety evaluation of a pesticide.

2. A well designed and conducted multigeneration study providing no evidence that the pesticide exerts a selective effect on repro-

duction or enhancement of general toxic effects should be given a high weighting towards establishing its safety.

3. The detection of effects in a multigeneration study may require further studies if the protocol has a limited ability for characterizing a specific effect.

4. The limited sensitivity of some end-points of a reproduction study needs to be borne in mind. Discrete responses such as pregnant or non-pregnant, "fertile" or "infertile" are quite insensitive, since objective discrimination between groups is governed by the same laws of statistical probability as are applicable to other low frequency events such as malformations.

5. Support studies such as examination of sperm motility and morphology may provide a sensitive end-point that can allow further characterization of effects observed in reproduction studies.

6. Histopathological examination of gonads performed in chronic toxicity studies may also provide valuable supplementary information.

8.3.4 Neurotoxicity studies

8.3.4.1 Delayed neurotoxicity

JMPR first reviewed feeding studies in hens, with subsequent examination of brain, spinal cord and sciatic nerves, in 1967 when dimethoate was evaluated [41]. In 1968, the first study using single doses in hens was reviewed, when dioxathion was evaluated [43]. The question of delayed neurotoxicity was first considered in 1974 [53] in response to requests from various countries for guidance on the introduction and use of the organophosphate leptophos. This was considered further at the 1975 JMPR, the report stating:

"A major toxicological problem long recognized to be associated with such organophosphate esters as tri-0-cresylphosphate (TOCP), and more recently brought to the attention of the Meeting in the evaluation of leptophos is that known commonly as 'delayed neurotoxicity' . . . The delayed neurotoxicity syndrome affects only certain animal species, including man. The most susceptible animal for laboratory bioassay procedures, the adult hen, is not susceptible before 3-4 months of age. While the adult hen is the animal of choice for laboratory testing, cats, dogs, calves, and sheep have been shown to be susceptible. Some sub-human primates and rodents are resistant to both the clinical and the histological lesions. In contrast, man has been shown to be highly susceptible to the syndrome, as suggested by studies where occurrences of paralysis have been reported . . . There are no known antidotes to delayed neurotoxicity, and recovery from ataxia is predominantly through development of collateral nerve pathways and physical therapy to develop muscles not served by affected nerves." [54, p. 11-12].

A certain degree of peripheral nerve regeneration also occurs, but regeneration is not observed in the central nervous system (CNS) axons. Therefore, the ataxia is clinically "irreversible" although the picture changes from a flaccid paralysis (peripheral nerve plus CNS lesions) to a spastic paralysis (CNS lesions only).

Reference has been made in some studies [14; 22; 104] to the induction of neurotoxicity by certain organophosphorus compounds used as pesticides and drugs. The dose administered in most experimental studies is high, and atropine has been used to protect animals from acute signs of poisoning to allow time for the neurotoxicity syndrome to develop. While atropine protects against the short-term acute cholinergic signs of poisoning,it is ineffective against delayed neurotoxicity occurring 8-14 days after treatment.

A key factor in the problem of delayed neurotoxicity, discussed by the 1975 Joint Meeting and endorsed by the 1976 [55] and 1978 [59] Meetings, is the dose response. "The Meeting concluded that delayed neurotoxicity appears to follow a dose-response relationship and that it is therefore possible to estimate a no-effect level following acute or chronic exposure in a susceptible species. With an adequate margin of safety an ADI for man can be allocated with a sufficient degree of assurance as far as pesticide residues in food are concerned." [54, p. 13].

The 1982 JMPR, in discussing acceptable protocols for pesticide toxicology studies, indicated that "multiple dosing (single oral doses, 21 days apart) was required for studies of delayed neurotoxicity of organophosphorus compounds." [67, p. 2].

The 1984 Meeting noted that:

"Some OPs (organophosphates) induce both acute reversible and delayed irreversible neurotoxicity; the latter relates to inhibition of another enzyme called neuropathy target esterase (NTE) [115]. Organophosphorus-delayed neurotoxicity is believed to be initiated by a two-step mechanism: a high level of NTE inhibition and 'aging' of the phosphoryl enzyme complex [105]."

"Inhibition of NTE within 24-48 hours after dosing correlates with the clinical and morphological effects of delayed neurotoxicity seen 10-20 days later. This test model was found to be valid for all OPs known to cause delayed neuropathy in man." [147].

The JMPR recommended that delayed neurotoxicity testing need not be done for monomethylcarbamates, phosphinates, or sulfonates. They also recommended that TOCP be used as a positive control only for OPs and that the NTE assay be included in the assessment of OPs [72].

The most recent comments on delayed neurotoxicity relate to the optical isomers of organophosphorus esters. The 1987 JMPR stated:

"Recent evidence suggests that when racemic mixtures of phosphonates are used in test animals, the optical isomers might show the same phosphonylating ability for NTE but the rates of aging might differ. Consequently only the optical isomer which forms an ageable protein-phosphonyl complex will cause delayed polyneuropathy. This was the case for EPN, an OP no longer in use. Therefore, whenever OPs are mixtures of optical isomers the delayed neurotoxic potential might depend on the chirality." [78, p. 11].

Two types of studies are generally conducted on chemicals suspected of being neurotoxic. The first is the use of a suitable sensitive species (usually the adult hen), where test substance is administered at two acute exposures (separated by 21 days) to atropine-protected animals at a level at or above the LD_{50} of the compound. Observations on body weight, ataxia, and signs of delayed neurotoxicity are made while the animals are alive. At termination, usually 42 days after the first dose, histopathological examination of the brain, spinal cord and proximal and distal sections of (usually) the sciatic nerve is performed. Data from this type of test suffer from two major drawbacks: the evaluation is often subjective, and a negative result cannot be graded. The second type of test is the determination of NTE activity [13; 105]. In its simplest form, this involves treatment of the adult hen with a single maximum tolerated dose of the test substance and subsequent assay of the brain enzyme after the time of peak inhibition but before substantial re-synthesis of new enzyme has occurred. The time of peak inhibition, which can be from 3 to 48 h post-dosing (and is determined by the pharmacokinetics of the compound), can often be assessed by observation of the time of onset of cholinergic signs. The threshold level of NTE inhibition at this early stage, which correlates with delayed neurotoxicity, is approximately 80%. No clinical signs are associated with an inhibition of 60% or less. When multiple determinations of NTE are made during chronic exposures, plateau levels are observed in 2-3 weeks. If inhibition of NTE in the brain and spinal cord is less than 50%, delayed neuropathy does not occur. However, inhibition of 60-70% in such studies might result in neuropathic sequelae as reported by some authors, while others state that the same threshold of NTE inhibition (70-80%) has to be reached in single and repeated exposures.

8.3.4.2 Acute neurotoxicity (acetylcholinesterase inhibition)

In 1967, the WHO Scientific Group on Procedures for Investigating Intentional and Unintentional Food Additives [169] noted that plasma and erythrocyte cholinesterase activities were markedly reduced by organophosphorus and carbamate pesticides. This Group also noted the absence of a correlation between blood cholinesterase levels and the signs and symptoms of toxicity. Thus cholinesterase levels in blood "may be useful as an indication of exposure to a substance with anti-cholinesterase activity, but not as an invariable guide to the degree of intoxication present or predicted" [169, p. 17-18]. The Group indicated that "although changes in blood cholinesterase levels may be helpful in toxicological studies, it is important that further research should be done to relate the indices used as closely as possible to the biochemical changes concerned in bringing about the toxic effects . . . " [169, p. 18].

Cholinesterase-inhibiting compounds have been evaluated at virtually every Joint Meeting. Until 1982, JMPR used inhibition of plasma cholinesterase, as well as erythrocyte and brain cholinesterase, for the purpose of establishing NOELs. In 1982, the status of cholinesterase activity as an indicator of anticholinesterase compound toxicity was reconsidered:

"In reviewing some organophosphorus and carbamate pesticides, the Meeting noted that previous JMPR reports have commented on, and made recommendations on the basis of, inhibition of plasma cholinesterase as a major criterion in the evaluation of some of these compounds. The present Meeting recognized that most organophosphorus compounds inhibit butyrylcholinesterase, known also as plasma cholinesterase or pseudocholinesterase, at concentrations lower than those at which they inhibit acetylcholinesterase found in erythrocytes and in nerve synapses.

"The function of plasma cholinesterase is not understood but it is known that it plays no role in cholinergic transmission, the physiological function which is impaired by anticholinesterases. On the other hand, acetylcholinesterase in erythrocytes, although playing no role in cholinergic transmission itself, reflects the acetylcholinesterase activity in nerve synapses, since the two enzymes are considered biochemically identical. Therefore, erythrocyte cholinesterase activity may be taken as an indicator of the biochemical effect of anticholinesterase pesticides." [67, p. 6].

A biologically significant reduction in erythrocyte cholinesterase is normally considered to be a reduction of >20% of pretest levels in the same animals in short-duration studies, or in concurrent controls in longer studies.

The 1988 Joint Meeting further considered the utility of plasma cholinesterase and erythrocyte and brain acetylcholinesterase measurements [79]. It noted that "the correlation between acetylcholinesterase inhibition in erythrocytes and in the nervous system is usually unknown" and indicated that "data on brain acetylcholinesterase inhibition are considered to be of greater value than those on erythrocytes in assessing the cholinergic effects of cholinesterases." The Meeting also noted, however, that in the absence of measurements of brain acetylcholinesterase, those of erythrocyte acetylcholinesterase serve as a better indicator of toxicity than those of plasma cholinesterase activity. It was noted that *in vitro* kinetic studies may be necessary for pesticides with anti-esterase activity. Results of these studies in different species may be combined with *in vivo* study findings to establish ADIs for these compounds.

JMPR has drawn attention to the methodology for measuring cholinesterase inhibition, stating that "the currently used methods for the determination of cholinesterase activity may lead to erroneous conclusions when applied to rapidly reversible cholinesterase inhibitions (e.g., *N*-methyl- and *N,N*-dimethylcarbamates). *In vitro* kinetic studies should be made to elucidate the nature of reversible inhibition reactions. The results obtained in *in vivo* studies should be interpreted cautiously until more satisfactory methods are available." [55, p. 11].

In 1983 [70], the problem of measurement of cholinesterase inhibition by carbamate pesticides was again addressed by JMPR. The report of this Meeting states "the Meeting noted that in the reports of several studies on carbamate pesticides, the method of determination of cholinesterase inhibition was inadequately reported and occasionally data were inconsistent with respect to dose and the degree of cholinesterase inhibition. Carbamates are considered to be reversible inhibitors of cholinesterase with a short duration of action. Because of the reversible inhibition of the enzyme by dilution, as would occur during the preparation of the assay, inhibition cannot be accurately measured. The Meeting stressed that in order to permit evaluation of cholinesterase inhibition by carbamates *in vivo*, special care is required in reporting all details of such studies." [70, p. 10]. Carbamate cholinesterase inhibition studies should utilize minimal dilution during the preparation of the assay, minimal incubation times and minimal times between blood sampling and assay (e.g., the Ellman method [28]).

8.3.4.3   Chronic neurotoxicity

The 1972 JMPR [50] noted the work of Murphy & Cheever [144], which reported modification of the electroencephalographic patterns in certain experimental animals following long-term exposure to low levels of cholinesterase-inhibiting compounds. The Meeting indicated that "insufficient information was available to permit any conclusion to be reached on the relationship of these studies to the toxicological assessment of cholinesterase-inhibiting compounds." [50, p. 8].

The 1974 Meeting [53] reiterated the desirability of determining the usefulness of electroencephalographic criteria for assessing the effects of cholinesterase-inhibiting pesticides. However, no further information or verification of this aspect of cholinesterase-inhibiting pesticide toxicity has become available to JMPR.

8.3.4.4   Pyrethroid-induced neurotoxicity

JMPR has evaluated data on pyrethroids during many meetings since 1965 [39; 47; 51; 61; 63; 66; 182]. Most pyrethroids can be divided into two classes: the T-syndrome (tremor) and the CS-syndrome (coreoathetosis-seizures). In general, alpha-cyanopyrethroids cause CS-syndrome neurotoxic effects, and other pyrethroids cause T-syndrome effects. The 1984 Meeting [73] noted that the neurotoxicity of pyrethroids originates from their primary action on the sodium channels of nerve membranes [123]. This interaction is reversible, as are the clinical signs of toxicity.

Morphological changes in peripheral nerves are produced as a secondary effect of the primary interaction only at doses close to the

LD_{50}. Therefore, considering the reversibility of pyrethroid neuro-toxicity and the high doses required to cause permanent secondary effects, the neurotoxicity of pyrethroids is not considered to be of great concern in the evaluation of pesticide residues in food.

8.3.4.5 Neurobehavioural toxicity

A recent WHO publication [175] on the Principles and Methods for the Assessment of Neurotoxicity Associated with Exposure to Chemicals stated the following:

"There is ample evidence of real and potential hazards of environ-mental chemicals for nervous system function. Changes or disturbances in central nervous function, many times manifest by vague complaints and alterations in behaviour, reflect on the quality of life; however, they have not yet received attention. Neurotoxicological assessment is therefore an important area for toxicological research. It has become evident, particularly in the last decade, that low-level exposure to certain toxic agents can produce deleterious neural effects that may be discovered only when appropriate procedures are used. While there are still episodes of large-scale poisoning, concern has shifted to the more subtle deficits that reduce functioning of the nervous system in less obvious, but still important ways, so that intelligence, memory, emotion, and other complex neural functions are affected. Information on neurobehaviour, neurochemistry, neurophysiology, neuroendocrinology, and neuropathology is vital for understanding the mechanisms of neuro-toxicity. One of the major objectives of a multifaceted approach to toxicological studies is to understand effects across all levels of neural organization. Such a multifaceted approach is necessary for confirmation that the nervous system is the target organ for the effect. Interdisciplinary studies are also necessary to understand the significance of any behavioural changes observed and thus to aid in extrapolation to human beings by providing specific neurotoxic pro-files. Concomitant measurements at different levels of neural organiz-ation can improve the validity of results."

Since the publication of this monograph, a number of protocols for neurobehavioural toxicity have been proposed for use [11]. However, the 1989 JMPR noted that the use of behavioural tests in laboratory animals has not been validated [183]. The meeting concluded: "This failure relates both to the inter-individual and intra-individual vari-ations in behaviour and the difficulty in quantifying these changes. In addition, the biochemistry, electrophysiological and morphological correlates of observed changes are often lacking." Although much has been written on behavioural teratology [158; 159], no data on this aspect of toxicology has been reviewed by JMPR. A discussion of the utility of these tests will be found in reference [174].

8.3.4.6   Principles

1. Delayed neurotoxicity appears to follow a dose-response relation-ship. Thus, with an adequate margin of safety an ADI can be allo-cated.

2. Delayed neurotoxicity testing should be conducted routinely for organophosphates. However, it need not be done for monomethyl-carbamates, phosphinates, or sulfonates.

3. TOCP is recommended as a positive control substance only for organophosphates.

4. The NTE assay should be included in the data base for organophos-phate evaluations.

5. Data on brain acetylcholinesterase are of greater value in safety assessment than are data on erythrocyte acetylcholinesterase.

6. Plasma cholinesterase (butyrylcholinesterase) inhibition is not considered to be an adverse toxicological effect.

8.3.5   Genotoxicity studies

The topic of mutagenicity (now generally referred to by the broader term, genotoxicity) and its relevance to the evaluation of the safety of pesticide residues has been repeatedly considered by JMPR. Most recently, the 1983 Meeting recognized the uncertainty of the associ-ation between mutagenic and carcinogenic activity, and indicated that data from long-term carcinogenicity studies must override any possible concerns raised by mutagenicity studies. In considering mutagenicity tests *per se*, the 1983 JMPR was unable to determine the relevance of the results of such tests to possible human health hazards. It there-fore indicated such data cannot be utilized directly in the assessment of the ADI [70].

A recent publication [5] surveying 222 chemicals tested in mice and rats (NCI/NTP bioassays) has indicated a strong association between structure/activity, mutagenicity in *Salmonella* strains, and the extent and sites of rodent tumourigenicity. When structure/activity and *Salmonella* tests were considered and utilized as an index of genotox-icity, the use of such an index indicated two groups of carcinogens: those that are genotoxic and those that are apparently non-genotoxic. In examining sites of action, some 16 tissues were susceptible to car-cinogenic effects with genotoxins only (accounting for 31% of the indi-vidual chemical/tissue reports), whereas the remaining 13 tissues were affected by both groups of carcinogens, the most frequently affected tissue being the mouse liver (24% of all individual chemical/tissue reports). Furthermore, chemicals active as carcinogens in both rats and mice, or in two or more tissues, showed a 70% correlation with positive *Salmonella* tests, whereas single species or single tissue carcinogens showed only 39% correlation. The study also confirmed that many *in vitro* genotoxins were not carcinogenic (possibly due to malabsorption, metabolism *in vivo*, or the supposedly greater sensitivity of the *in vitro* tests). Mouse liver-specific carcinogens were also *Salmonella* positive in only 30% of the cases, indicating that mouse liver tumour induction may be mechanistically independent of interaction of the test chemical with DNA.

These results support the position that rodent carcinogenicity tests are required for all pesticide evaluations (see section 8.3.4.1), since without such studies it cannot be determined that a pesticide is a trans-species, multiple-tissue rodent carcinogen.

8.3.5.1 Principles

1. Mutagenicity is utilized only as supplementary information in the weight-of-the-evidence determination for carcinogenicity.

2. Mutagenicity tests, especially mammalian *in vivo* tests, which are indicative of compound-induced alterations in DNA are of value in assisting in the determination of the mechanism of action of some carcinogens.

3. Genotoxicity testing is also potentially useful in the prediction of the risk of heritable defects.

4. Protocols that are sensitive, practical, and predictive of heritable human risk remain to be developed.

8.3.6 Immunotoxicity studies

8.3.6.1 Background

In 1967, progressive haemolytic anaemia was observed in monkeys exposed to dieldrin [41]. However, it was not recognized at the time that this anaemia resulted from antibodies produced in the animal which were directed against dieldrin bound to the erythrocytes [89]. The 1976 JMPR "noted the first observation in a group of animals of a pesticide (pirimicarb) causing a haemolytical reaction which might be of an immuno-reactive nature. In the case observed, the phenomenon occurred only with relatively high doses in a closed, inbred colony of dogs. However, it is possible that, by prolonged and constant use of such a pesticide, hypersensitivity may be built up which could eventually lead to an immunological reaction of a haematological or other nature." [55, p. 14]. In 1978, JMPR [59] again considered pirimicarb, and noted that haemolytic changes occurred in a second strain of dogs but not in monkeys or in rodent species. The effect was therefore considered to be species specific.

8.3.6.2   Current position

Immunotoxicology has been defined as the discipline concerned with the study of events that can lead to undesired effects as a result of the interaction of test substances with the immune system. These undesired effects may be a consequence of:

- direct and/or indirect action of the test substance (and/or its biotransformation product) on the immune system;

- an immunologically-based host response to the compound and/or its metabolites;

- host antigens modified by the compound or its metabolite(s).

Zbinden [181] has indicated that chemicals may affect the immune system immediately and preferentially, but they may also act either by injury to other organs or by creating a general deterioration of the health of the animal, resulting in a secondary effect on the immune system. Consequently, as with any aspect of toxicology, immunotoxicology must be considered in the light of all available toxicity data and not as an entity independent of other factors.

In mammals the primary lymphoid tissues comprise the thymus, spleen, lymph nodes, bone marrow and diffuse lymphoid tissues associated with the gastrointestinal and respiratory systems [117; 165]. Progenitor cells produced in the bone marrow and other lymphoid tissues undergo maturation in early life via residence in the thymus to produce the T-cell series (which are mainly responsible for cell-mediated immunity), and via development in peripheral lymphoid tissues to become members of the B-cell series, which form the basis of humoral (antibody-mediated) immunity. Throughout life, the development of immune reactions and defenses involves interactions between several types of T- and B-cells and soluble factors produced by early stages of these cells, phagocytic cells, and polymorphs.

Chemically-induced immune alterations may be detectable from pathological changes (quantitative and qualitative) in lymphoid organs. Thus, changes in the weight of the thymus, spleen, and lymph nodes, combined with histopathological changes in these organs can be important in assessing the potential immunotoxicity of a chemical. Furthermore, examination of mucosa-associated lymphoid tissue (e.g., Peyer's patches) may indicate immunotoxic potential. Examination of bone marrow is essential in any immunotoxic assessment, as is consideration of the resistance to infection of the living animal.

Atrophy and lymphocytic depletion in the thymic cortex, hypoplasia or hypercellularity of the paracortical areas of the lymph node, changes in the numbers of lymphoid follicles, changes in germinal centres and plasma cells in lymph nodes and the spleen, and the size and cellularity of the marginal zone of the spleen may all be indicative of immunotoxicity. However, other factors also induce some of these effects (e.g., thymic atrophy due to stress or weight loss) [165].

Haematological studies of serial blood samples for total and differential leucocyte counts and platelet numbers can provide a potential indicator of certain autoimmune processes. Similarly, measurements of body temperature and serum chemistry to determine cortisol and fibrinogen levels may suggest consequences of certain types of immunotoxicity [121].

The recognition that an increased tumour incidence (especially lymphomas) can be associated with immunosuppression indicates that the immune system may be involved in controlling neoplastic changes. This involvement is supported by *in vivo* evidence of tumour immunogenicity (e.g., transplant rejection; lymphoid cell transfer experiments), by the promising use of monoclonal antibodies as therapeutic agents in cancer therapy, and by many laboratory demonstrations of cellular and humoral responses to neoplasms.

A number of agents (e.g., tricothecene mycotoxins), known to occur as contaminants in food, can be shown to affect the immune system of laboratory animals. These mycotoxins (nivalenol, deoxynivalenol, etc.), which are unaffected by heating or baking, occur on cereal crops grown in temperate climates. Information on the potential of pesticide residues to interact with such immunosuppressive agents would be of value in the safety assessment of pesticides.

It is becoming apparent that immune dysfunctions induced by test substances sometimes have severe and diverse health effects ranging from autoimmune diseases or hypersensitivity reactions to the possible induction of cancer. In the past, this area has received little attention because of the lack of basic knowledge of suitable test methods. The complexity of the mechanisms of action of the immune system makes it difficult to decide on appropriate studies. Some potential probably exists for the general identification of immunotoxicants from standard toxicological protocols, but full identification of immunotoxicity is likely to require further ancillary studies. The development of additional methods relevant to the safety assessment of pesticide residues is to be encouraged in the hope that sets of tests, suitably validated, will permit evaluation of this important aspect of toxicology. A collaborative study, sponsored by the IPCS and CEC, is currently underway to examine and validate test methodologies for the assessment of immunotoxicity.

8.3.6.3   Principles

1. Immune dysfunctions induced by test substances can result in serious health effects and should be considered in the evaluation of pesticide residues in food.

2. Validation of a tiered approach to immunotoxicity tests relevant to safety assessment is to be encouraged.

8.3.7   Absorption, distribution, metabolism, and excretion

8.3.7.1   Background

The meeting held in 1961 to consider Principles Governing Consumer Safety in Relation to Pesticide Residues [32] indicated that the procedures to be followed in generating data for the safety evaluation of a pesticide "must be determined by . . . its toxicological and biochemical actions, as they are discovered during the progress of the investigation." The report also cited the second and fifth JECFA reports [31; 33], indicating that the procedures detailed in these reports should be followed when a new pesticide is being investigated.

The second JECFA report addressed biochemical and other special investigations. It indicates that "the aspects of metabolic and biochemical activity that might be profitably studied include the route and rate of absorption of the test material, the levels of storage in tissues and the subsequent fate of the stored material. Studies of the metabolism of the material, together with the identification of the metabolites, might be extended to include balance experiments, in which an attempt is made to account for the administered dose as metabolites excreted or material stored in the body" [31, p. 13]. The report indicated that studies should be performed initially at high dose levels and later they should be extended to investigate lower dose levels. It also indicated that examination of enzyme processes and studies using pharmacodynamic techniques may be useful in specific cases.

The 1963 JMPR stated that "it is important to know whether a substance is absorbed, its distribution in the body after absorption, its mechanism of action including its influence on enzyme systems, how it is metabolized, and the routes of final elimination. The toxicity of a pesticide may be altered at any of these stages." [35, p. 8].

A WHO Scientific Group in 1967 also indicated the importance of metabolism studies, stating that:

"The detailed study of metabolism at the molecular level has been applied to many problems and this has special relevance to toxicology. Modification of substances in the course of their metabolism may significantly affect their toxicity; chemicals may alter enzyme activity and some substances may stimulate the production of metabolizing enzymes. Hence for a full understanding of the effects of a chemical on biological systems, it is necessary to have as much knowledge as possible about the relationship between the chemical (and its derivatives) and the complex pattern of enzymes in living organisms." [169, p. 4].

In the section of the report that addressed enzyme studies, the Scientific Group stated:

"It has become more and more apparent that, among the mechanisms of action of toxic substances, those of a biochemical nature are of prime importance. In this connection, the basic enzyme systems are certainly among the first sites of action to merit careful study, since their inhibition often constitutes the causal biochemical lesion that determines, at least in part, the nature of toxic effects." [169, p. 14].

In 1975, JMPR [54] re-emphasized the principle that tissue distribution and the mode and rate of metabolism and excretion can profoundly influence the toxicity of a compound. It noted, however, that such data were usually based on single-dose studies. In proposing the need for multiple-dose studies, the Meeting noted that biliary excretion, with the potential for enterohepatic circulation, and the problems of distribution and storage of highly lipophilic substances in fat deposits, as well as potential accumulation of slowly metabolized compounds, would not be adequately addressed by single-dose studies.

8.3.7.2 Current position

In discussing doses in toxicity studies and extrapolation to humans, the 1987 JMPR indicated that comparative metabolism of the test material in the experimental animal and man were basic to the choice of dose levels [78]. The Meeting recognized the rarity of such data and the ethical problems involved in obtaining the required data in the required sequence (i.e. experiments in man prior to completion of all animal studies). In addition, the following points were made:

1. "The processes involved in absorption, distribution, biotransformation, and excretion are dependent upon many factors, including physico-chemical properties, extent of protein binding, bioavailability, and dose. Some of these processes are saturable. Products of biotransformation may be formed at different rates and in different quantities, or by different pathways at high doses (e.g., 2-phenylphenol) . . . It is valid to extrapolate animal data to man only if the biotransformation pathways of the chemical are identical or very similar between species, and if the doses do not exceed the capacity of the pathways being compared. If this capacity is exceeded, different metabolites may be produced.

2. "Kinetic data are useful in the design of studies and in the interpretation and extrapolation of the data. For example, if the test material is not absorbed, the need for one or more long-term studies would be obviated.

3. "Extrapolation of animal data to man may be compromised by differences between species in the movement of the chemical after absorption. For example, the administration of high doses of certain chemicals may result in increased enterohepatic circulation of the chemical and/or its metabolites. This is an important system in the rat, but less so in man.

4. "The proper design of definitive long-term studies should be based on comparative data on absorption, distribution, biotransformation, excretion, and appropriate kinetic considerations of the test substance." [78, p. 3-4].

Some explanation of specific points in the above quote are required to clarify the intent of JMPR. Point 1 emphasizes the importance of obtaining comparative metabolism and pharmacokinetic data in humans and the species in which a toxic effect is observed. Although in the absence of such data it is assumed that biotransformation in humans and the test species is similar, only comparative metabolic studies can confirm the validity of the extrapolation. In point 2, species differences regarding absorption should be considered. The variability in gut microflora between species and the possible effects of intestinal breakdown products require consideration. Similarly, the use of kinetic data to determine whether a "steady state" has been achieved (i.e. the achievement of a state of equilibrium between intake and excretion) is important in protocol design.

From the above discussion, it is apparent that data on pharmacokinetics, pharmacodynamics, biotransformation, and studies on enzymes are basic to many considerations in toxicology. Since toxic activity depends on the interaction of a chemical and a target site (or sites) in the intact animal, some knowledge of the identity and quantity of the material and/or its metabolites reaching the target site is needed. The 1986 JMPR stressed the importance of understanding the mechanisms that result in the expression of toxicity. It noted that: "Current knowledge of mechanisms of toxicity is limited, but there is already a sufficient understanding in some cases to permit better design, performance, and interpretation of toxicological studies. Mechanistic studies are therefore encouraged, since a knowledge of mechanism of action is likely to result in a more rational assessment of the risk to man." [76, p. 2].

The material absorbed may be the administered chemical(s), or it may be metabolites and/or reaction products of the administered chemical. Variations in absorption occur because of species differences (especially when specialized transport mechanisms are involved in absorption, such as those encountered with metals), differences in intestinal flora (discussed extensively in reference [176]), age, nutritional status, dietary fibre content, and factors affecting motility. The identity of the absorbed material may also differ markedly from that administered, due to acid-mediated hydrolysis in the stomach, breakdown by gastrointestinal enzymes (e.g., splitting of peptides), chemical reactions between food components (e.g., nitrosamine formation by reaction between nitrite and secondary amines in the stomach), and the activity of the intestinal flora. Secondary absorption may also occur, arising from biliary excretion and subsequent reabsorption of the excreted material, either in its original excreted form or following hydrolysis in the intestine.

Information about the site of absorption of the test material is also important, since this may alter the overall metabolism and thus the toxicological profile of the test substance. If absorption occurs in the buccal cavity, the oesophagus, or the stomach, it is likely to be distributed widely throughout the body in the form in which it is absorbed. If absorption is from the small intestine, the transportation of the absorbed material will be via the hepatic portal system to the liver. Within the liver, it may be metabolized, resulting in distribution of metabolites rather than of parent compound. This factor is of major importance when considering routes of exposure other than those by the oral route. Resolution of these potential problems can be achieved by adequate pharmacokinetic and metabolic data.

Once absorbed from the gastrointestinal tract, distribution depends on a variety of factors, which may differ between and within species. For example, the age of the animal, the rate of metabolism, the degree of previous exposure, and the amount and rate of blood flow through different organs may all affect the eventual distribution of the absorbed material. The distribution and, ultimately, the concentration at the receptor level, is greatly influenced by the ability of the chemical to penetrate biological membranes such as the placenta, glomerular membrane, and the blood/brain barrier. This, in turn, is primarily a function of lipophilicity, molecular size, and extent of ionization (pK_a).

The metabolism of the absorbed material depends on an equally wide range of variables:

- the degree of enzyme development is dependent on age;

- enzymes may vary between species, both qualitatively and quantitatively;

- Michaelis-Menten kinetics indicate that saturation of enzyme systems may occur at some level, either increasing the importance of secondary mechanisms of metabolism or resulting in greater plasma levels of parent compound;

- the site of metabolic activity may differ among species (e.g., microbial metabolism in the rodent stomach, which is not observed in humans, primates, or dogs);

- the rate of metabolism may differ within and between species and between different tissues and cells;

- interaction among test substances may occur, or metabolism may be affected by other test substances (e.g., enzyme inhibition, stimulation, or induction);

- duration of exposure (acute or chronic) may modify the rate and pathways of metabolism.

Both the route and rate of excretion of a test substance may vary between species. The pharmacokinetic parameters of clearance and biological half-life are considered to be indicators of the potential for accumulation. However, rapid elimination of a chemical and its metabolites clearly does not necessarily equate to a lack of toxicity.

Use of radioactive labelling or heavy isotope techniques provides data on absorption, distribution, and excretion. These studies assist in the identification of sites of covalent binding, and are virtually indispensable in the study of metabolism and pharmacokinetics. Data from such studies, in conjunction with analytical determinations of excreted products, provide the basis for determining the probable metabolic pathways for administered compounds. It must be remembered that in interpreting studies involving radiolabelling techniques, consideration must be given to the site of the label on the molecule and the stability (mobility) of the radiolabel. Thus, an organic molecule containing several different ring structures may require multiple studies, with radiolabelling at different sites in the molecule, to ensure the determination of all metabolic products.

The above list of factors is incomplete, but nevertheless serves to indicate the complexity of the problems associated with studies of absorption, distribution, metabolism, and excretion of a test substance. For useful publications covering these issues, the reader is referred to the comprehensive texts which have been published on the subject (e.g., reference [107]).

8.3.7.3 Principles

1. Studies on absorption, distribution, metabolism, and excretion are essential in the evaluation of the safety of a pesticide. These studies provide a foundation for the interpretation of all other toxicology studies.

2. Ethically conducted comparative metabolic and pharmacokinetic studies in humans and animal test species may permit more accurate extrapolation of animal data to humans.

9. EVALUATION OF DATA

9.1 Extrapolation of Animal Data to Humans

The objective of the safety evaluation of pesticide residues in food is to determine the maximum daily intake of the pesticide that will not result in adverse effects at any stage in the human lifespan. Since, in the majority of cases, data on humans are inadequate to permit such a determination, effects observed in other species must be extrapolated to humans. Ideally, data on comparative pharmacokinetics, metabolism, and mechanism of action should be utilized in the extrapolation. However, such data are not available in the majority of cases. The use of relevant biomarkers of exposure and effect such as the formation of adducts to DNA or blood proteins like haemoglobin in humans and test animals may also be useful in the extrapolation across species. Further research in this area is to be encouraged.

Three basic approaches are now generally used in the extrapolation of the results of studies in experimental animals to humans: the use of safety factors, the use of pharmacokinetic extrapolation (widely used in the safety evaluation of pharmaceuticals), or the use of linear low-dose extrapolation models.

JMPR has not utilized the third approach (the use of linear low-dose extrapolation models). A number of these models have been used to determine the "virtually safe dose" (VSD) of carcinogens for humans. One major drawback of these models is the lack of consideration of many of the biological factors which should be taken into account. Furthermore, the various mathematical models available (Probit, Wiebel, etc.), when applied to the same data, can result in VSD values which vary by orders of magnitude. There is no agreement among toxicologists on the "best" mathematical model available today, nor on whether these mathematical models have any biological meaning at all.

Pharmacokinetic extrapolation requires human pharmacokinetic data, which are rarely available for pesticides. The method involves a comparison of pharmacokinetics in human and experimental animals. The relative sensitivity of receptor sites must also be taken into consideration.

The JMPR approach has generally been limited to the first of the three approaches, that is the use of safety factors. These are applied to the NOAEL determined from the experimental animal data, or preferably, from data in humans, if available.

9.2 Safety Factors

9.2.1 Background

The 1963 JMPR adopted the commonly used empirical approach for the extrapolation of data to man, i.e. "the maximum no-effect dietary level obtained in animal experiments, expressed in mg/kg body weight per day, was divided by a 'factor', generally 100." [35, p. 11]. This concept appears to have been adopted from the report of the second JECFA Meeting which states that ". . . a dosage level can be established that causes no demonstrable effects in the animals used. In the extrapolation of this figure to man, some margin of safety is desirable to allow for any species differences in susceptibility, the numerical differences between the test animals and the human population exposed to the hazard, the greater variety of complicating disease processes in the human population, the difficulty of estimating the human intake, and the possibility of synergistic action among food additives." [31, p. 17]. The Committee then stated that the 100-fold margin of safety applied to the maximum ineffective dose (expressed in mg/kg body weight per day) was believed to be an adequate factor.

The 1965 JMPR [36] discussed the concept of the acceptable daily intake and safety factors. It noted that the 100-fold factor could be modified according to circumstances (e.g., reduction to 10 or 20 fold when human data are available or in the case of well-studied organophosphates).

The 1966 JMPR indicated that when a temporary ADI was allocated, the margin of safety applied to the NOAEL derived from experimental animal data should be increased [38]. These principles were applied by the 1966 Joint Meeting when establishing a temporary ADI for pyrethrin (safety factor of 250) [39].

A WHO Scientific Group considered safety factors in 1967 [169]. This Group noted that safety factors could be varied and described circumstances where increased safety factors should be used. These included toxicological data gaps and when it was necessary to establish temporary ADIs. Decreasing the margin of safety was proposed when pertinent biological data indicates uniform species response, when the initial effect is clear-cut and reversible, or when cholinesterase inhibition or adaptive liver enlargement is the initial effect. Otherwise a 100-fold safety factor was considered to be a useful guide.

The 1968 JMPR [42] indicated that, where human data comprised the basis for the NOAEL used in determining the ADI, a smaller safety factor might be utilized. This statement was amplified by the 1969 JMPR [44] to include human biochemical as well as toxicological data as justification for reducing safety factors.

The 1975 JMPR, in addressing the question of safety factors in toxicological evaluation, stated that:

"It should be emphasized that the magnitude of the margin of safety applied in each individual case is based on the evaluation of all available data. In consideration of any information that gives rise to particular concern, the magnitude of the margin of safety will be increased. Where the data provide an assurance of safety, the magnitude may be decreased. Therefore, it is impossible to recommend fixed rules for the margin of safety to be applied in all instances." [54, p. 9].

In 1977, the JMPR "wished to clarify the situation regarding safety factors in arriving at ADIs for man. The establishment of the ADI for man is not a simple arithmetic exercise based on the no-effect level, as the safety factor may vary widely from one compound to another. Although safety factors are determined empirically, they are dependent on the nature of the compound, the amount, nature and quality of the toxicological data available, the nature of the toxic effects of the compound, whether the ADI or TADI for man is established, and the nature of any further data required." [57, p. 4].

During a discussion on general principles used by the JMPR, the 1984 Meeting [72] stressed the degree of uncertainty that accompanies a toxicological evaluation, and stated:

"The use of variable safety factors by the JMPR in the estimation of ADI values reflects this uncertainty, and underlines the complexity of assessing the human health hazards of pesticides. No hard and fast rules can be made with regard to the magnitude of this safety factor, since many aspects have to be considered, such as species differences, individual variations, incompleteness of available data, and a number of other matters such as considerations of the fact that pesticide residues may be ingested by people of all ages throughout the whole life-span, that they are eaten by the sick and the healthy as well as children, and that there are wide variations in individual dietary patterns." [72, p. 3].

The original concept of the use of 100-fold safety factors was based on interspecies and intraspecies variations [114]. Included in this consideration were variations between strains, provision for sensitive human population sub-groups, and possible synergistic effects due to exposure to more than one chemical.

The 100-fold safety factor can be viewed as two 10-fold factors, one for inter- and one for intra-species variability [111]. While these safety factors appear, on the basis of experience, to provide adequate margins of safety in the extrapolation of data to man, they may, of course, be questioned. Some experimental support for safety factors was published by Dourson & Stara [26] in 1983. This paper also proposed an additional 10-fold factor for extrapolating sub-chronic data, and for converting lowest-observed-adverse-effect levels to NOAELs (factors of 1-10, depending upon the severity and concern raised by the observed effect). Additional clinical and epidemiological research may improve the characterization of the variation in response within the human population to various pesticides and may allow a more accurate determination of safety factors.

9.2.2   Principles

When determining ADIs, the 100-fold safety factor is used as the starting point for extrapolating animal data to man and may be modified in the light of the data that are available and the various concerns that arise when considering these data. Some of these are given below:

1. When relevant human data are available, the 10-fold factor for inter-species variability may not be necessary. However, relatively few parameters are studied in man in the assessment of pesticide safety, and data on oncogenicity, reproduction, and chronic effects are rarely available. Thus, even if the parameter measured in humans is the same as the most sensitive adverse effects measured in the experimental animal (e.g., erythrocyte cholinesterase depression), uncertainty still remains with respect to the potential effects on other parameters. This usually necessitates an increased safety factor. Consequently, JMPR rarely utilizes safety factors as low as 10-fold.

2. The quality of the data supporting the NOAELs determined in the animal experiments (and also in human experiments) influences the choice of the safety factor. Unfortunately, toxicity studies are rarely perfect in all respects. While a study may serve to answer a basic question, the degree of certainty with which the question is answered may be reduced by, for example, increased mortality in all groups in an oncogenicity study, resulting in marginally-acceptable data being available at the termination of the study. When a request for a repeat study is not fully justified, an increased safety factor may be utilized under such circumstances.

3. The quality of the total data base may affect the choice of safety factor. Significant data deficits may warrant an increased safety factor due to increased uncertainty.

4. The type and significance of the initial toxic response may alter the safety factor. Thus a response which is reversible may result in a reduced safety factor.

5. The limited numbers of animals used in oncogenicity studies limits the sensitivity of the study in the identification of a threshold dose. When evidence of neoplasia has been identified, safety factors may be increased depending on the available ancillary data and the establishment of an NOAEL.

6. The shape of the dose/response curve (in those cases where data are adequate to permit derivation of such a curve) may also be considered in assessing safety factors.

7. Metabolic considerations may influence the choice of the safety factor. Thus, saturation of metabolic pathways resulting in toxic manifestations, biphasic metabolic patterns, and data on comparative metabolism may all affect the magnitude of the safety factor.

8. Knowledge of the comparative mechanism of toxic action in experimental animals and man may influence the choice of safety factor.

Several of the factors cited above may apply in the consideration of any one compound. Certain factors may serve to increase and others to decrease the choice of the final safety factor. Therefore, it must be stressed that the total weight of evidence has to be considered in determining the appropriate safety factor to be used and that the determination of safety factors must be considered on a case-by-case basis.

9.3 Allocating the ADI

9.3.1 Background

The FAO/WHO Joint Meeting on Principles Governing Consumer Safety in Relation to Pesticide Residues indicated that the assessment of the amount of pesticide to which man can be exposed daily for a lifetime, without injury, was the primary aim of toxicological investigations. The Meeting indicated that "when the (toxicological) investigations are completed, it is possible, by the use of scientific judgement, to name the acceptable daily intake." [32, p. 9]. The meeting also defined the ADI as follows:

"The daily dosage of a chemical which, during an entire lifetime, appears to be without appreciable risk on the basis of all the facts known at the time. 'Without appreciable risk' is taken to mean the practical certainty that injury will not result even after a lifetime of exposure. The acceptable daily intake is expressed in milligrams of the chemical, as it appears in the food, per kilogram of body weight (mg/kg)." [32, p. 5].

The first JMPR adopted this definition and discussed the concept of the ADI. The Meeting stated that the following information should be available in order to arrive at an ADI:

(a) "the chemical nature of the residue. Pesticides may undergo chemical changes and are frequently metabolized by the tissues of plants and animals which have been treated with them. Even when a single chemical has been applied, the residues may consist of a number of derivatives with distinct properties, the exact nature of which may differ in animals and plants and in different crops and products.

(b) the toxicities of the chemicals forming the residues from acute, short-term and long-term studies in animals. In addition, knowledge is required of the metabolism, mechanism of action and possible carcinogenicity of residue chemicals where consumed.

(c) A sufficient knowledge of the effects of these chemicals in man." [35, p. 6].

The Meeting also noted that the identity of the food bearing the chemical should theoretically be immaterial; that the ADI was an expression of opinion, which carried no guarantee of "absolute" safety; that new knowledge or data could always lead to re-evaluation of an ADI; and that JMPR would confine itself to proposing a single set of ADI figures for pesticides. Finally, the Meeting stated that "The proposed levels (of ADIs) could normally be regarded as acceptable throughout life; they are not set with such precision that they cannot be exceeded for short periods of time." [35, p. 7] (see section 9.3.3).

Although the ADI can be exceeded for short periods of time, it is not possible to make generalization on the duration of the time frame which may cause concern. The induction of detrimental effects will depend upon factors which vary from pesticide to pesticide. The biological half-life of the pesticide, the nature of the toxicity, and the amount by which the exposure exceeds the ADI are all crucial.

The large safety factors generally involved in establishing an ADI also serve to provide assurance that exposure exceeding the ADI for short time periods is unlikely to result in any deleterious effects upon health. However, consideration should be given to the potentially acute toxic effects that are not normally considered in the assessment of an ADI.

The principles discussed above were adopted by subsequent Joint Meetings but, as would be expected, have been further developed with time. Thus the 1968 JMPR [42] indicated that metabolites would, under certain conditions, be considered to be included in the ADI. Generally, if the metabolites in food commodities are qualitatively and quantitatively the same as those observed in laboratory test species, the ADI would apply to the parent compound as well as to metabolites. If the metabolites are not identical or not present at the same order of magnitude, separate studies on the metabolites may be necessary. When one or several pesticides are degradation products of another pesticide, a single ADI may be appropriate for the pesticide and its metabolites, e.g., oxydemeton-methyl, demeton-S-methyl sulfone and demeton-S-methyl [183].

In 1973, when considering the accuracy with which ADIs or TADIs could be estimated, JMPR recommended that ADIs should be expressed numerically using only one significant figure [52]. The use of more than one significant figure might be taken to imply a greater degree of accuracy than that which can be achieved when assessing the hazard from the wide range of factors that influence toxicity.

9.3.2   Temporary ADIs

Use of the TADI, first proposed by the Scientific Group on Procedures for Investigating Intentional & Unintentional Food Additives [169], was adopted by JMPR in 1966. Criteria were set that had to be met prior to the establishment of the TADI. These included the consideration of each chemical on its own merits, the establishment of the

TADI for a fixed period (usually 3-5 years), and the subsequent review of original and new data prior to the expiration of the provisional period.

The establishment of a TADI has always been accompanied by a requirement for further work by a specified date and by the application of an increased safety factor. The 1972 JMPR considered the course of action to be taken if requested data were not forthcoming and indicated that, under these circumstances, the TADI would be withdrawn. It emphasized, however, that such an action "did not necessarily indicate a potential health hazard, but only that insufficient information is available at the time of review to permit the Meeting to state with reasonable certainty that there is no likelihood of adverse effects on health resulting from ingestion over a prolonged period." [50, p. 7].

In 1986 [76], JMPR indicated that the previously utilized terms "Further work or information required" or "Further work or information desirable" were being replaced, the former by the statement "Studies without which the determination of an ADI is impracticable", and the latter by the statement "Studies which will provide information valuable to the continued evaluation of the compound." These new statements not only reflect the actual work performed by JMPR much more clearly than the previous terms "Required" and "Desirable", but they also reflect the Meeting's increasing reluctance to allocate temporary ADIs as well as the desire to continue the evaluation of a compound even after an ADI has been allocated.

In 1988 [79], JMPR recommended that TADIs should not be allocated for new compounds and that an ADI should not be allocated in the absence of an adequate data base. The Meeting intended that monographs be published for all chemicals which are reviewed, regardless of whether an ADI is allocated, and that data requirements will be clearly specified for those chemicals with an inadequate data base.

The concept of the "conditional acceptable daily intake", adopted by the 1969 JMPR [44], was limited to those compounds for which the use was at that time considered essential but for which the toxicological data base was incomplete. This concept, which is unacceptable, has been abandoned.

9.3.3   Present position

The minimum data base normally utilized in determining an ADI comprises short-term feeding studies, long-term feeding studies, carcinogenicity studies, multigeneration reproduction studies, teratogenicity studies, and acute and repeated exposure metabolic, toxicokinetic, and toxicodynamic data. Where deemed necessary, additional special studies may also be required, e.g., genotoxicity studies.

The NOAEL from the most appropriate study divided by the appropriate safety factor determines the ADI. The lowest NOAEL is not necessarily the basis for the ADI (see section 8.2.1). Thus, even though the NOAEL from a chronic toxicity study may be less than that from a reproduction study, the latter may serve as the basis for assessing the ADI, because of the potential use of a higher safety factor (see section 9.2). On this basis, the entire age range of the population is normally covered by the ADI. The present procedure therefore provides an acceptable margin of safety to the entire population for those pesticides with complete data bases. The advantage of providing separate ADIs for different age (or physiological) groups of the population, would therefore be limited to indicating those groups who may be in a reduced-risk category, rather than indicating those at increased risk.

A document entitled "Guidelines for Predicting Dietary Intake of Pesticide Residues" was published by WHO in 1989 [177]. This document provides guidance on the prediction of the dietary intake of residues of a pesticide for the purpose of comparison with the ADI allocated by JMPR. The document recommends a step-wise approach to predicting intake, considering average consumption of the treated commodities and a number of factors (such as processing, variations in residues level with time and the percentage of a given commodity that is treated) that usually have the effect of providing a more accurate prediction of real pesticide residue intake. An example of dietary intake calculations for a hypothetical pesticide is given in Chapter 3 of "Guidelines for Predicting Dietary Intake of Pesticide Residues."

10. EVALUATION OF MIXTURES

10.1 Introduction

Survey data indicate that residues of more than one pesticide may be detected in food. This gives rise to concern over the possibility of unanticipated interactions between such residues leading to adverse toxicological effects. There is, of course, a virtually unlimited number of combinations of pesticides on various crops. There is also a very large number of combinations of foods containing pesticide residues.

10.2 Background

The possibility of pesticide interaction was recognized as early as 1961 when the FAO/WHO Meeting on Principles Governing Consumer Safety in Relation to Pesticide Residues recognized that "different pesticides and other chemicals are often absorbed simultaneously during occupational use, or in food, by man or animals" [32, p. 10]. The first JMPR [35] also noted the possibility of interactions between chemicals in discussions on the shortcomings of the ADI. It was indicated that ADI values were calculated on the assumption that the diet was contaminated by a single residue, hence additive and synergistic effects were not considered. An extensive review of the significance of interactions of pesticides was performed by the 1967 JMPR [40]. The 1981 Joint Meeting gave further consideration to interaction between pesticide residues and concluded that:

1. "Not only could pesticides interact, but so could all compounds (including those in food) to which man could be exposed. This leads to unlimited possibilities, and there is no special reason why the interactions of pesticide residues (which are at very low levels) should be highlighted as being of particular concern;

2. "Very little data on these interactions are available;

3. "The data obtained from acute potentiation studies are of little value in assessing ADIs for man." [62, p. 12].

10.3 Principle

The consideration of mixtures of residues does not require any change in the general principles for estimating ADIs. However, there is a need for further data on interactions of pesticides with each other and with other common contaminants of food (e.g., metals, mycotoxins) to ensure that, at the very low levels of pesticide exposure likely to occur via dietary residues, and over the prolonged time periods involved in such human exposure, no adverse effects are likely to occur.

11. RE-EVALUATION OF PESTICIDES

In 1961, the Meeting on Consumer Safety in Relation to Pesticide Residues stated that "of necessity early views of the amount (ADI) will be estimated and subject to revision as experience accumulates" [32, p. 9]. Thus, from its inception, the provisional nature of the ADI has been recognized [35]. The 1965 Meeting [36] re-examined the 37 pesticides reviewed in 1963 [35]. Changes in the ADIs were instituted for 16 of these pesticides, based on additional information that had become available.

The need for a full re-evaluation of the toxicity data base on some pesticides was identified by the 1981 JMPR [65], based on concerns over the validity of previously submitted data (see section 5.1). The first of these re-evaluations was undertaken in 1982 [64]. The development of new methods for investigating toxicity has also caused concern in relation to pesticides for which ADIs have been established [52].

The use of the TADI [40] ensures re-evaluation of the data base pertaining to specific compounds, since one of the criteria for setting a TADI is that identified data are required for evaluation by a specific time. However, a more systematic method of re-evaluation has been suggested such as the automatic re-evaluation of chemicals reviewed more than 10 years previously [72, p. 8].

Establishing a priority order for the re-evaluation of compounds requires input from a number of sources including the Codex Committee on Pesticide Residues (CCPR). This Committee has initiated this process for pesticides evaluated prior to 1976 [30].

12. BIOTECHNOLOGY

Biotechnology comprises a number of different approaches to pest control. Three areas are of emerging concern: the production of chemicals of biological origin with pest-control activity (e.g., hydroprene); the use of microbial pest control agents (e.g., bacteria, fungi, viruses, and protozoa); and the development and use of genetically altered (bioengineered) organisms for specific purposes.

At the present time, JMPR has no experience with these types of pest-control products other than limited experience with biologically derived chemicals (e.g., pyrethrin). The following comments are therefore proposals leading to approaches which may be feasible in assessing the safety of such products.

First, with regard to the so-called "biorational" products, these chemicals are derived from or are synthesized to be identical to naturally occurring pesticidal agents. The fact that they are naturally occurring does not necessarily mean that they are safe. Thus, such chemicals should be investigated in the same way as other synthetic chemicals used as pesticides. In certain instances, it is possible that justification for reducing the necessary toxicological data base may exist.

In dealing with microbial pest-control agents and bioengineered organisms, two factors are of primary importance to human health - the infectivity of the residual organism and the ability of the organism to produce toxins which occur as residues. In the case of viruses, their ability to incorporate into the cell genome should also be considered.

The determination of the safety of microorganisms should follow a tiered approach, tier 1 being the determination of infectivity and toxicity based on acute administration. If measurable survival of the microorganisms in the test animal is still apparent several days after administration, short-term feeding studies may be deemed to be appropriate. If exotoxins are produced by the microorganisms, then the toxin should be isolated, identified, and subjected to tests similar to those for any other chemical utilized as a pesticide. Similarly, if an endotoxin is produced and there is evidence that this material could be released, the endotoxin should also be subjected to standard toxicology testing, as required for other chemical pesticides. In the event of both endo- and exo-toxin having potential access to humans or to domestic animals, consideration should be given to simultaneous administration of the two compounds in toxicity studies. If circumstances exist that would indicate the possibility of waiving any of the routine toxicity tests, scientifically supported evidence indicating the absence of need for such tests must be provided.

13. SPECIAL CONSIDERATIONS FOR INDIVIDUAL CLASSES OF PESTICIDES

13.1 Organophosphates - Ophthalmological Effects

In 1972, JMPR noted published reports suggesting that certain ophthalmological effects may be induced by exposure to some organophosphate insecticides [50]. Insufficient information was available at that time to permit a toxicological assessment of the significance of the reports. In 1979, additional reports were considered by JMPR [52]. The Meeting again concluded that insufficient information was available to permit an evaluation. No additional information has been considered by JMPR.

13.2 Organophosphates - Aliesterase (carboxylesterase) Inhibition

The 1967 JMPR [40], in considering interactions between pesticides, noted that "some of the aliesterases are more sensitive than the cholinesterases to inhibition by certain organophosphorus compounds [83]. Furthermore, those organophosphates that are more active as aliesterase inhibitors than as cholinesterase inhibitors appear to be the most effective in potentiating the toxicity of other organophosphates [27]. Also, the aliesterases participate in the detoxication of many of the organophosphates and probably other chemicals to which humans may be exposed. For these reasons, it is suggested that consideration be given to the use of no-effect levels for aliesterase inhibition rather than no-effect levels for cholinesterase inhibition, as a basis for estimating the daily acceptable intakes of those organophosphorus insecticides to which the aliesterase systems are more sensitive than are the cholinesterases" [40, p. 38].

In 1972, JMPR noted that short-term feeding studies demonstrated the fact that in the case of many organophosphate pesticides, inhibition of liver and serum carboxylesterases was a more sensitive parameter than inhibition of cholinesterases [122; 151]. However, it noted that "the physiological significance of carboxylesterase inhibition is still unknown" [50, p. 8]. Since carboxylesterase inhibition appears to be a factor in potentiation, JMPR indicated the desirability of further work in this area. The 1974 Meeting [53] reiterated the need for information to determine the usefulness of aliesterase inhibition in assessing the safety of organophosphate compounds.

Carboxylesterases mainly hydrolyze aliphatic esters, but their substrate specificity is not absolute. They can also hydrolyze aromatic esters at measurable rates. There is evidence for marked variation in humans, which is genetically determined. Since there is such variability, yet no data on the toxicological significance of these relatively non-specific enzymes, they are unlikely to be used to determine NOAELs in the evaluation of organophosphorus compounds. It should, however, be noted that some organophosphate impurities are potent carboxylesterase inhibitors and hence markedly potentiate the toxicity of pesticides that are detoxified by these enzymes (e.g., malathion).

13.3 The Need for Carcinogenicity Testing of Organophosphates

In 1986, JMPR noted that organophosphate compounds tend not to show genotoxicity *in vivo* or to induce carcinogenic responses in laboratory animals [76]. It was recommended that careful evaluation of all available data should be performed to determine whether carcinogenicity tests are required for individual organophosphate pesticides. It is also recommended that the possible structure-activity relationships of the non-phosphate ester moiety of the pesticide should be considered.

13.4 Ocular Toxicity of Bipyridilium Compounds

The pyridilium herbicides diquat and paraquat were first reviewed by JMPR in 1970 [77]. The studies on diquat demonstrated the induction of lens opacities in rats, dogs, and cows. Studies on paraquat, for the same duration and at the same dose levels as for diquat, did not demonstrate ocular effects in any species tested.

Additional data on both compounds were evaluated in 1972 [51]. At that time, it was demonstrated that prolonged administration of diquat was required to induce cataracts. The type of cataract induced differed structurally from those observed due to physical or disease processes. Again, no evidence of compound-related ocular damage was noted in rats or mice treated with paraquat.

In 1977, additional data on diquat showed that although the incidence of cataracts was no higher than that of control animals, an earlier appearance was observed [58]. Because the data base for paraquat had been generated by Industrial Biotest Laboratories, most studies of this chemical were repeated. These repeat studies were evaluated by the 1986 JMPR [77]. No cataracts were induced in a one year study in dogs or in a long-term feeding study in mice. Cataracts were observed in Fisher (but not Wistar) rats in long-term studies. Microscopic examination of these cataracts showed that, in contrast to diquat-induced cataracts, there was a close similarity to age-related cataracts in control animals. There is, therefore, some evidence that paraquat may cause some ophthalmological toxicity, even though this has only been observed in one strain of one species, and even then the lesions noted are similar in type to age-related lesions. However, it would be advisable to perform careful ophthalmological studies on any bipyridilium compounds that may be developed as future herbicides.

13.5 Goitrogenic Carcinogens

A probable mechanism for this class of compounds is described below.

Diets low in iodine, causing chronic iodine deficiency in experimental animals, lead to hypertrophy, hyperplasia, and follicular cell neoplasia of the thyroid gland and pituitary gland adenomas [6; 8; 80; 81; 145]. These effects have also been observed with subtotal thyroid-ectomy [24], splenic transplantation of thyroid tissue [10], and the transplantation of pituitary tumours that secrete thyroid-stimulating hormone (TSH) [24; 90; 148]. The fact that none of these experimental techniques introduced exogenous agents, other than transplanted tissue, into the animal's internal environment indicated that the causative oncogenic mechanism must reside within the animal and must be mediated through the intimate interrelationship of the pituitary and thyroid glands.

This led to a concept, subsequently supported with experimental data, of a negative feedback system which maintained a homeostatic balance between the pituitary and thyroid gland secretions. Later, the hypothalamus was added to this system when it was discovered that it exerted some control over pituitary gland secretions. Subsequent research indicated that, while the hypothalamus is essential to normal pituitary and thyroid gland functioning, the receptors residing within the pituitary/thyroid axis are of primary importance in controlling thyroid and pituitary hormonal balance [86; 97]. Disturbance of this balance has significant physiological and morphological effects on the glands as well as on the well-being of the animal [118].

Exogenous physical and chemical agents can also induce thyroid/pituitary hypertrophy, hyperplasia, and neoplasia by causing hormonal imbalance [9; 102; 180]. The chemical goitrogens were first discovered in animal and human food items [15; 88; 149]. Since then many chemically defined substances have been reported to induce thyroid/pituitary hypertrophy, hyperplasia, and, after prolonged exposure, neoplasia. Radioactive iodine and x-rays can produce the same effects [17; 25; 96; 98]. The mechanisms by which these substances and the non-agent experimental techniques produce their pharmacological (goitrogenic) and neoplastic effects are well known, even though the precise triggering event for the transformation from hyperplasia to neoplasia is still uncertain [9; 85; 87]. The most common mechanisms are interference with the thyroid iodide transport system or inter-ference with peroxidases essential to the synthesis and secretion of competent thyroid hormone [15; 18; 95; 138; 149; 156].

The sequence of events triggered by this interference is also well understood. As the circulation of competent thyroid hormone (TH) is reduced, the receptors in the hypothalamus and pituitary gland receive a signal for secretion of TSH. Receptors within the thyroid receive, through TSH, a signal for increased TH production and secretion and the gland responds, at first, with functional hypertrophy [86; 97]. Thus far these events may remain within the normal operation of the feedback system. At this stage, if the cause of the thyroid hormone deficiency is removed or corrected, the circulation of competent TH increases to a critical level and TSH secretion is reduced. As homeostasis is reestab-lished, the thyroid gland returns to normal. However, under conditions of chronic TH deficiency and the failure of the feedback mechanism to restore hormonal balance, both glands continue to respond to their respective signals and enter hypertrophic and hyperplastic states. The pituitary continues to secrete TSH, to which the thyroid responds, but the thyroid cannot signal for TSH shut off because of its inability to secrete competent TH. Eventually this relationship results in hormonal imbalance that induces thyroid gland follicular cell neoplasia and frequently pituitary gland neoplasia.

The hypothesis that thyroid/pituitary hormonal imbalance is the oncogenic mechanism is supported by evidence that follicular cell neoplasia can be prevented by the simultaneous administration of goitrogens and thyroid hormone. This has been demonstrated with thiouracil [9] and thiourea [143], two members of a class of potent goitrogens. The pharmacological effects, hypertrophy and hyperplasia, are reversible upon removal of the goitrogenic stimulus [4; 9; 85; 106; 140; 153]. Furthermore, NOELs have been demonstrated in several species, for both the goitrogenic and neoplastic effects of thyroid function inhibitors. These facts coupled with evidence that treatment of human hypothyroidism with goitrogens is without appreciable risk of thyroid neoplasia [92], support the concept of a threshold for goitrogen-induced thyroid follicular cell and pituitary neoplasia [137; 138].

The weight-of-evidence indicates that goitrogens occupy an unusual nitch in oncogenesis in that:

- their pharmacological effects and mechanisms of action are reasonably well understood;

- their pharmacological effects are reversible;

- thresholds, NOELs, and NOAELs can be established for their pharmacological and neoplastic effects;

- pituitary and thyroid neoplasia potentially induced by thyroid inhibitors can be prevented by supplying experimental animals with competent thyroid hormones during treatment with goitrogens;

- a certain degree of thyroid inhibition is accommodated for prolonged periods within the homeostatic control limits of the normally functioning feedback mechanism;

- long-term exposure to excessive TSH is required before hormonal imbalance induces thyroid follicular cell neoplasia.

Increased TSH secretion is the ultimate common mediator of thyroid follicular proliferative lesions induced by goitrogens, its level is moderated by a feedback mechanism, and its neoplasm-inducing potential is subject to mechanisms demonstrating threshold effects. Laboratory animal data demonstrate that there is an ordered linkage of steps: thyroid blockade, continuous TSH release, thyroid hypertrophy/hyperplasia, modularity, and adenoma/carcinoma. They also show that a threshold for an early step automatically becomes a threshold for the whole chain of steps. These characteristics should be a major consideration when assessing the human oncogenic potential of thyroid-function inhibitors.

REFERENCES

1. ALDRIDGE, W.N. (1986) The biological bases and measurement of thresholds. Annu. Rev. Pharmacol. Toxicol., 26: 39-58.

2. AMES, B.N. (1983) Dietary carcinogens and anticarcinogens. Oxygen radicals and degenerative diseases. Science, 221: 1256.

3. ANDERSON, M.E., CLEWALL, H.J., GARGAS, M.L., SMITH, F.A., & REITZ, R.H. (1987) Physiologic based pharmacokinetics and the risk assessment process for methylene chloride. Toxicol. appl. Pharmacol., 87: 185-206.

4. ARNOLD, D.L., KREWSKI, D.R., JUNKINS, D.B., MCGUIRE, P.F., MOODIE, C.A., & MUNRO., I.C. (1983) Reversibility of ethyl-enethiourea-induced thyroid lesions. Toxicol. appl. Pharmacol., 67: 264-273.

5. ASHBY, J. & TENNANT, R.W. (1988) Chemical structure, Salmonella mutagenicity and extent of carcinogenicity as indicators of genotoxic carcinogenesis amongst 222 chemicals tested in rodents by the US NCI/NTP. Mutat. Res., 204: 17-215.

6. AXELROD, A.A. & LEBLOND, C.P. (1955) Induction of thyroid tumors in rats by a low iodine diet. Cancer, 8: 339-367.

7. BARSHNECHT, T.G., NAISMITH, R.W., & KORNBULL, D.J. (1987) Variations in the standard protocol design of the rat hepatocyte DNA repair assay. Cell Biol. Toxicol., 3: 193-208.

8. BIELSCHOWSKY, F. (1953) Chronic iodine deficiency as a cause of neoplasia in thyroid and pituitary of aged rats. Br. J. Cancer, 7(2): 203-213.

9. BIELSCHOWSKY, F. (1955) Neoplasia and internal environment. Br. J. Cancer, 9: 80-116.

10. BRACHETTO-BRIAN, D. & GRINBERG, R. (1951) Histological development of intrasplenic thyroid autografts in thyroidectomized rats. Rev. Soc. Argent. Biol., 27: 199-204.

11. BURIN, G.J. (1988) Report of FIFRA Scientific Advisory Panel on Neurotoxicity, Washington, DC, US Environmental Protection Agency, Office of Pesticide Programmes.

12. BYRNE, G. (1987) Conviction of Bruening. Science, 24: 1004.

13. CAROLDI, S. & LOTTI, M. (1982) Neurotoxic esterase in peripheral nerve: assay, inhibition and rate of resynthesis. Toxicol. appl. Pharmacol., 62: 498-501.

14. CAVANAGH, J.B. (1973) Peripheral neuropathy caused by toxic agents. CRC Crit. Rev. Toxicol., 2: 365.

15. CHESNEY, A.M., CLAWSON, T.A., & WEBSTER, B. (1928) Endemic goitre in rabbits. I. Incidence and characteristics. Bull. John Hopkins Hosp., 43(5): 261-277.

16. CHRISTIAN, M.S. (1986) A review of multigeneration studies. J. Am. Coll. Toxicol., 5: 161-180.

17. CHRISTOV, K. (1978) Radiation-induced thyroid tumours in infant rats. Radiat. Res., 73(2): 330-339.

18. CHRISTOV, K. & STOICHKOVA, N. (1977) Cytochemical localization of peroxidase activity in normal proliferating and neoplastic thyroid tissue of rats. An ultrastructural study. Acta histochem., 58: 5275-5289.

19. CLAYSON, D.B. (1974) Bladder carcinogenesis in rats and mice: Possibility of artifacts. J. Natl Cancer Inst., 52: 1685-1689.

20. CLEGG, D.J. & WANDELMAIER, F. (1987) An investigation into the desirability of the inclusion of a second litter per generation in rat multigeneration studies. In: Greenhalgh, R. & Roberts, T.R., ed. Pesticide science and biotechnology, Boston, Blackwell Scientific Publications, pp. 549-552.

21. CIOMS (1982) Proposed international guidelines for biomedical research involving human subjects, Geneva, Council for International Organizations of Medical Sciences.

22. DAVIES, D.R. (1963) Neurotoxicity of organophosphorus compounds. In: ' Koelle, G.B., ed. [Handbook of experimental pharmacology], Supplement 15, Berlin, Springer Verlag, pp. 860-882 (in German).

23. DEMPSTER, A.P., SELWYN, M.D., & WEEKS, B.J. (1983) Combining historical and randomized controls for assessing trends in proportions. J. Am. Stat. Assoc., 78: 221-227.

24. DENT, J.N., GODSDEN, E.L., & FURTH, J. (1956) Further studies on induction and growth of thyrotropic pituitary tumors in mice. Cancer Res., 16: 171-174.

25. DONIACH, I. (1950) The effect of radioactive iodine alone and in combination with methylthiouracil and acetylaminofluorene upon tumor production in rat thyroid gland. Br. J. Cancer, 4(2): 223-234.

26. DOURSON, M.L. & STARA, J.F. (1983) Regulatory history and experimental support of uncertainty (safety) factors. Regul. Toxicol. Pharmacol., 3: 224-238.

27. DUBOIS, K.P. (1987) The comparative inhibitory action of organic phosphates on several esterases and arudases and the relationship of esterase inhibition to phosphate potentiation. Unpublished paper presented to the Gordon Research Conference on Toxicology and Safety Evaluation, Meriden, New Hampshire, August 1967.

28. ELLMAN, G.I., COURTNEY, K.D., ANDRES, V., Jr, & FEATHERSTONE, R.M. (1967) A new and rapid colorimetric determination of acetylcholinesterase activity. Biochem. Pharmacol., 7: 88-95.

29. FAO (1959) Report on the Meeting of the FAO Panel of Experts on the Use of Pesticides in Agriculture held in Rome, 6-13 April 1959, Rome, Food and Agriculture Organization of the United Nations. (Meeting Report No. 1959/3).

30. FAO (1989) Report of the Twentieth Session of the Codex Committee on Pesticide Residues, Rome, Food and Agriculture Organization of the United Nations, Codex Alimentarius Commission (Alinorm 89/24).

31. FAO/WHO (1958) Procedures for the testing of intentional food additives to establish their safety for use. Second Report of the Joint FAO/WHO Expert Committee on Food Additives, Geneva, World Health Organization (FAO Nutrition Meeting Report Series, No. 17; WHO Technical Report Series, No. 144).

32. FAO/WHO (1962a) Principles governing consumer safety in relation to pesticide residues, Geneva, World Health Organization (FAO Plant Production and Protection Division Report, No. PL/1961/11; WHO Technical Report Series, No. 240).

33. FAO/WHO (1962b) Evaluation of the carcinogenic hazard of food additives. Fifth Report of the Joint FAO/WHO Expert Committee on Food Additives, Geneva, World Health Organization (FAO Nutrition Meeting Report Series, No. 29; WHO Technical Report Series, No. 220).

34. FAO/WHO (1964a) Report of the First Meeting of the FAO Working Party on Pesticide Residues, Rome, Food and Agriculture Organization (Meeting Report No. PL/1963/16).

35. FAO/WHO (1964b) Evaluation of the toxicity of pesticide residues in food. Report of a Joint FAO/WHO Meeting of the FAO Committee on Pesticides in Agriculture and the WHO Expert Committee on Pesticide Residues, Geneva, World Health Organization (FAO Meeting Report No. PL/1963/13; WHO/Food Add./23).

36. FAO/WHO (1965a) Evaluation of the toxicity of pesticide residues in food. Report of the Second Joint Meeting of the FAO Committee on Pesticides in Agriculture and the WHO Expert Committee on Pesticide Residues, Geneva, World Health Organization (FAO Meeting Report No. PL/1965/10; WHO/Food Add./26.65).

37. FAO/WHO (1966) Report on the Second Meeting of the FAO Working Party on Pesticide Residues, Rome, Food and Agriculture Organization of the United Nations (Meeting Report No. PL/1965/12).

38. FAO/WHO (1967a) Pesticide Residues in Food. Joint Report of the FAO Working Party on Pesticide Residues and the WHO Expert Committee on Pesticide Residues, Geneva, World Health Organization (FAO Agricultural Studies No. 73; WHO Technical Report Series, No. 370).

39. FAO/WHO (1967b) Evaluation of some pesticide residues in Food, Geneva, World Health Organization (FAO/PL:CP/15; WHO/Food Add./67.32).

40. FAO/WHO (1968a) Pesticide residues. Report of the 1967 Joint Meeting of the FAO Working Party and the WHO Expert Committee, Geneva, World Health Organization (FAO Meeting Report No. PL:1967/M/11; WHO Technical Report Series, No. 391).

41. FAO/WHO (1968b) 1967 Evaluations of some pesticide residues in food: The monographs, Geneva, World Health Organization (FAO/PL:1967/M/11/1; WHO/Food Add./68.30).

42. FAO/WHO (1969a) Pesticide residues in food. Report of the 1968 Joint Meeting of the FAO Working Party of Experts on Pesticide Residues and the WHO Expert Committee on Pesticide Residues, Geneva, World Health Organization (FAO Agricultural Studies No. 78; WHO Technical Report Series, No. 417).

43. FAO/WHO (1969b) 1968 Evaluations of some pesticide residues in food: The monographs, Geneva, World Health Organization (FAO/PL:1968/M/9/a; WHO/Food Add./69.35).

44. FAO/WHO (1970a) Pesticide residues in food. Report of the 1969 Joint Meeting of the FAO Working Party of Experts on Pesticide Residues and the WHO Expert Group on Pesticide Residues, Geneva, World Health Organization (FAO Agricultural Series, No. 84; WHO Technical Report Series, No. 458).

45. FAO/WHO (1970b) 1969 Evaluations of some pesticide residues in food: The monographs, Geneva, World Health Organization (FAO/PL: 1969/M/17/1.

46. FAO/WHO (1971a) Pesticide residues in food. Report of the 1970 Joint Meeting of the FAO Working Party of Experts on Pesticide Residues and the WHO Expert Committee on Pesticide Residues, Geneva, World Health Organization (FAO Agricultural Studies No. 87; WHO Technical Report Series, No. 474).

47. FAO/WHO (1971b) 1970 Evaluations of some pesticide residues in food: The monographs, Geneva, World Health Organization (AGP:1970/M/12/1; WHO/Food Add./71.42).

48. FAO/WHO (1972a) Pesticide residues in food. Report of the 1971 Joint Meeting of the FAO Working Party of Experts on Pesticide Residues and the WHO Expert Committee on Pesticide Residues, Geneva, World Health Organization (FAO Agricultural Studies No. 88; WHO Technical Report Series, No. 502).

49. FAO/WHO (1972b) 1971 Evaluations of some pesticide residues in food: The monographs, World Health Organization (WHO Pesticide Residues Series, No. 1).

50. FAO/WHO (1973a) Pesticide residues in food. Report of the 1972 Joint Meeting of the FAO Working Party of Experts on Pesticide Residues and the WHO Expert Committee on Pesticide Residues, Geneva, World Health Organization (FAO Agricultural Studies No. 90; WHO Technical Report Series, No. 525).

51. FAO/WHO (1973b) 1972 Evaluations of some pesticide residues in food: The monographs, Geneva, World Health Organization (WHO Pesticide Residues Series, No. 2).

52. FAO/WHO (1974) Pesticide residues in food. Report of the 1973 Joint Meeting of the FAO Working Party of Experts on Pesticide Residues and the WHO Expert Committee on Pesticide Residues, Geneva, World Health Organization (FAO Agricultural Studies No. 92; WHO Technical Report Series, No. 545).

53. FAO/WHO (1975) Pesticide residues in food. Report of the 1974 Joint Meeting of the FAO Working Party of Experts on Pesticide Residues and the WHO Expert Committee on Pesticide Residues, Geneva, World Health Organization (FAO Agricultural Studies No. 97; WHO Technical Report Series, No. 574).

54. FAO/WHO (1976) Pesticide residues in food. Report of the 1975 Joint Meeting of the FAO Working Party of Experts on Pesticide Residues and the WHO Expert Committee on Pesticide Residues, Geneva, World Health Organization (FAO Plant Production and Protection Series, No. 1; WHO Technical Report Series, No. 592).

55. FAO/WHO (1977a) Pesticide residues in food. Report of the 1976 Joint Meeting of the FAO Panel of Experts on Pesticide Residues and the Environment and the WHO Expert Group on Pesticide Residues, Geneva, World Health Organization (FAO Food and Nutrition Series, No. 9; FAO Plant Production and Protection Series, No. 8; WHO Technical Report Series, No. 612).

56. FAO/WHO (1977b) 1976 Evaluations of some pesticide residues in food: The monographs, Rome, Food and Agriculture Organization of the United Nations (AGP:1976/M/14).

57. FAO/WHO (1978a) Pesticide residues in food - 1977. Report of the Joint Meeting of the FAO Panel of Experts on Pesticide Residues and Environment and the WHO Expert Committee on Pesticide Residues, Rome, Food and Agriculture Organization of the United Nations (FAO Plant Production and Protection Paper 10 Rev.).

58. FAO/WHO (1978b) Pesticide residues in food - 1977 Evaluations: The monographs, Rome, Food and Agriculture Organization of the United Nations (FAO Plant Production and Protection Paper 15 Sup.).

59. FAO/WHO (1979) Pesticide residues in food - 1978. Report of the Joint Meeting of the FAO Panel of Experts on Pesticide Residues in Food and Environment and the WHO Expert Group on Pesticide Residues, Rome, Food and Agriculture Organization of the United Nations (FAO Plant Production and Protection Paper 15).

60. FAO/WHO (1980a) Pesticide residues in food - 1979. Report of the Joint Meeting of the FAO Panel of Experts on Pesticide Residues in Food and the Environment and the WHO Expert Group on Pesticide Residues, Rome, Food and Agriculture Organization of the United Nations (FAO Plant Production and Protection Paper 20).

61. FAO/WHO (1980b) Pesticide residues in food - 1979 Evaluations: The monograph, Rome, Food and Agriculture Organization of the United Nations (FAO Plant Production and Protection Paper No. 20 Sup.).

62. FAO/WHO (1981a) Pesticide residues in food - 1980. Report of the Joint Meeting of the FAO Panel of Experts on Pesticide Residues in Food and the Environment and the WHO Expert Group on Pesticide Residues, Rome, Food and Agriculture Organization of the United Nations (FAO Plant Production and Protection Paper 26).

63. FAO/WHO (1981b) Pesticide residues in food - 1980 Evaluations: The monographs, Rome, Food and Agriculture Organization of the United Nations (FAO Plant Production and Protection Paper 26 Sup.).

64. FAO/WHO (1981c) Evaluation of certain food additives. Twenty-fifth Report of the Joint FAO/WHO Expert Committee on Food Additives, Geneva, World Health Organization (WHO Technical Report Series, No. 669).

65. FAO/WHO (1982a) Pesticide residues in food - 1981. Report of the Joint Meeting of the FAO Panel of Experts on Pesticide Residues in Food and the Environment and the WHO Expert Group on Pesticide Residues, Rome, Food and Agriculture Organization of the United Nations (FAO Plant Production and Protection Paper 37).

66. FAO/WHO (1982b) Pesticide residues in food - 1981 Evaluations: The monographs, Rome, Food and Agriculture Organization of the United Nations (FAO Plant Production and Protection Paper 42).

67. FAO/WHO (1983a) Pesticide residues in food - 1982. Report of the Joint Meeting of the FAO Panel of Experts on Pesticide Residues in Food and the Environment and the WHO Expert Group on Pesticide Residues, Rome, Food and Agriculture Organization of the United Nations (FAO Plant Production and Protection Paper 46).

68. FAO/WHO (1983b) Pesticide residues in food - 1982 Evaluations: The monographs, Rome, Food and Agriculture Organization of the United Nations (FAO Plant Production and Protection Paper 49).

69. FAO/WHO (1983c) Evaluation of certain food additives and contaminants. Twenty-seventh Report of the Joint FAO/WHO Expert Committee on Food Additives, Geneva, World Health Organization (WHO Technical Report Series, No. 696 and corrigenda).

70. FAO/WHO (1984) Pesticide residues in food - 1983. Report of the Joint Meeting of the FAO Panel of Experts on Pesticide Residues in Food and the Environment and the WHO Expert Group on Pesticide Residues, Rome, Food and Agriculture Organization of the United Nations (FAO Plant Production and Protection Paper 56).

71. FAO/WHO (1985a) Pesticide residues in food - 1983 Evaluations: The monographs, Rome, Food and Agriculture Organization of the United Nations (FAO Plant Production and Protection Paper 61).

72. FAO/WHO (1985b) Pesticide residues in food - 1984. Report of the Joint Meeting on Pesticide Residues, Rome, Food and Agriculture Organization of the United Nations (FAO Plant Production and Protection Paper 62).

73. FAO/WHO (1985c) Pesticide residues in food - 1984 Evaluations: The monographs, Rome, Food and Agriculture Organization of the United Nations (FAO Plant Production and Protection Paper 67).

74. FAO/WHO (1986a) Pesticide residues in food - 1985. Report of the Joint Meeting of the FAO Panel of Experts on Pesticide Residues in Food and the Environment and a WHO Expert Group on Pesticide Residues, Rome, Food and Agriculture Organization of the United Nations (FAO Plant Production and Protection Paper 68).

75. FAO/WHO (1986b) Pesticide residues in food - Evaluations 1985: Part II - Toxicology, Rome, Food and Agriculture Organization of the United Nations (FAO Plant Production and Protection Paper 72/2).

76. FAO/WHO (1987a) Pesticide residues in food - 1986. Report of the Joint Meeting of the FAO Panel of Experts on Pesticide Residues in Food and the Environment and a WHO Expert Group on Pesticide Residues, Rome, Food and Agriculture Organization of the United Nations (FAO Plant Production and Protection Paper 77).

77. FAO/WHO (1987b) Pesticide residues in food - 1986 Evaluations: Part II - Toxicology, Rome, Food and Agriculture Organization of the United Nations (FAO Plant Production and Protection Paper 78/2).

78. FAO/WHO (1987c) Pesticide residues in food - 1987. Report of the Joint Meeting of the FAO Panel of Experts on Pesticide Residues in Food and the Environment and a WHO Expert Group on Pesticide Residues, Rome, Food and Agriculture Organization of the United Nations (FAO Plant Production and Protection Paper No. 84).

79. FAO/WHO (1988) Pesticide residues in food - 1988. Report of the Joint Meeting of the FAO Working Party of Experts on Pesticide Residues and the WHO Expert Committee on Pesticide Residues, Rome, Food and Agriculture Organization of the United Nations (FAO Plant Production and Protection Paper 92).

80. FORTNER, J.G., GEORGE, P.A., & STERNBERG, S.S. (1958) The development of thyroid cancer and other abnormalities in Syrian hamsters maintained on an iodine deficient diet. Surg. Forum, 9: 646-650.

81. FORTNER, J.G., GEORGE, P.A., & STERNBERG, S.S. (1960) Induced and spontaneous thyroid cancer in the Syrian (Golden) hamster. Endocrinology, 66: 364-376.

82. FOX, T.R. & WATENABE, P.G. (1985) Detection of a cellular oncogene in spontaneous liver tumors of $B6C1F_1$ mice. Science, 228: 596-597.

83. FRAWLEY, J.P. (1965) Synergism and antagonism in research in pesticides, New York, Academic Press, p. 73.

84. GEMS (1985) Guidelines for the study of dietary intakes of chemical contaminants, Geneva, World Health Organization, Global Environmental Monitoring System (WHO Offset Publication No. 87).

85. GILMAN, A.G. & MURAD, F. (1975) Thyroid and antithyroid drugs. In: Goodman, L.S. & Gilman, A.G., ed. The pharmacological basis of therapeutics, 5th ed., New York, MacMillan Publishing Company, pp. 1398-1422.

86. GOODMAN, H.M. & VAN MIDDLESWORTH, L. (1980) The thyroid gland. In: Mountcastle, V.B., ed. Medical physiology, Saint-Louis, Missouri, Mosby, Vol. 2, pp. 1495-1518.

87. GREEN, W.I. (1978) Mechanisms of action of anti-thyroid compounds. In: Werner, S.C. & Ingbar, S.H., ed. The thyroid, New York, Harper and Row, pp. 77-87.

88. GRIESBACH, W.E., KENNEDY, T.H., & PURVES, H.D. (1945) Studies on experimental goitre. VI. Thyroid adenomata in rats on brasse seed diets. Br. J. exp. Pathol., 26: 18.

89. HAMILTON, H.E., MORGAN, D.P., & SIMMONS, A. (1978) A pesticide (dieldrin) induced immunohaemolytic anemia. Environ. Res., 17: 155-164.

90. HARAN-GHERA, N., PULLAR, P., & FURTH, J. (1960) Induction of thyrotropin-dependent thyroid tumours by thyrotropes. J. Endocrinol., 66: 694-701.

91. HARDEN, M.S., SCHULER, R.L., BURG, J.R., BOOTH, G.M., HAZELDEN, K.P., MACKENZIE, K.M., PICCIRILLO, V.J., & SMITH, K.N. (1987) Evaluation of the Chernoff/Kavlock test for developmental toxicity. Teratog. Carcinog. Mutagen., 7(1): 1-128.

92. HAYES, W.J. (1982) Fungicides and related compounds. In: Pesticides studies in man, Baltimore, Maryland, Williams and Wilkins, p. 603.

93. HENRY, J.B., ed (1979) Todd-Sanford-Davidson's clinical diagnosis and management, Philadelphia, Pennsylvania, W.B. Saunders Co.

94. HEALTH AND WELFARE CANADA (1973) The testing of chemicals for carcinogenicity, mutagenicity and teratogenicity, Ottawa, Health and Welfare Canada, pp. 137-185.

95. HILL, R.N., ERDREICH, L.S., PAYNTER, O.E., ROBERTS, P.A., ROSENTHAL, S.L., & WILKINSON, C.F. (1989) Review - thyroid follicular cell carcinogenesis. Fundam. appl. Toxicol., 12: 629-657.

96 HINDAWI, A.I. & WILSON, C.M. (1965) The effects of irradiation on the function and survival of rat thyroid. Clin. Sci., 28: 555-571.

97. HINKLE, P.M. & GOH, K.B.C. (1982) Regulation of thyrotropin-releasing hormone receptors and response by L-triiodothyronine in dispersed rat pituitary cell cultures. Endocrinology, 110: 1725-1731.

98. HOLM, L.E., (1980) Thyroid treatment and its possible influence on occurrence of malignant tumors after diagnostic 131I. Acta radiol. oncol., 19(6): 455-459.

99. HUGHES, D.H., BRUCE, R.C., HART, R.W., FISHBEIN, L., GAYLOR, D.W., SMITH, J.M., & CARLTON, W.W. (1983) A report on the Workshop on Biological and Statistical Implications of the EDO1 Study and Related Databases. Fundam. appl. Toxicol., 3: 129-136.

100. IARC (1986) In: Gart, J.J., Krewski, D., Lee, P.N., Tarone, R.E., & Wahrendorf, J., ed. The design and analyses of long-term animal experiments. Statistical methods in cancer research, Volume III, Lyon, International Agency for Research on Cancer (IARC Scientific Publications No. 79).

101. IARC (1987) Preamble to IARC Monograph Programme on the Evaluation of Carcinogenic Risk to Humans, Lyon, International Agency for Research on Cancer.

102. ISRAEL, M.S. & ELLIS, I.R. (1960) The neoplastic potentialities of mouse thyroid under extreme stimulation. Br. J. Cancer, 14: 206-211.

103. IOANNIDES, C.V., LEEM, P.Y., & PARKE, D.V. (1984) Cytochrome P 448 and the activation of toxic chemicals and carcinogens. Xenobiotica, 14: 119.

104. JOHNSON, M.K. (1975) The delayed neuropathy caused by some organophosphorous esters: Mechanism and challenge. CRC Crit. Rev. Toxicol., 3: 289-316.

105. JOHNSON, M.K. (1982) The target for initiation of delayed neurotoxicity by organophosphorus esters: biochemical studies and toxicological applications. Rev. Biochem. Toxicol., 4: 141-212.

106. JULL, J.W. (1976) Endocrine aspects of carcinogenesis. In: Chemical carcinogens, Washington, DC, American Chemical Society, pp. 52-82 (ACS Monograph No. 173).

107. KATZUNG, B.G. (1987) Basic and clinical pharmacology, 3rd ed., Norwalk, Connecticut, Appicton and Lange.

108. KHERA, S. (1984) Maternal toxicity: a possible factor in foetal toxicity in mice. Teratology, 29: 411-416.

109. KHERA, K.S. (1985) Maternal toxicity: a possible etiological factor in embryofetal death and foetal malformations of rodent, rabbit species. Teratology, 31: 129-153.

110. KHERA, K.S. (1987) Maternal toxicity in humans and animals: effects on foetal development and criteria for their detection. Teratog. Carcinog. Mutagen., 7: 287-295.

111. KLAASSEN, C.D. (1986) Principles of toxicology. In: Klaassen, C.D., Amdur, M.O., & Doull, J., ed. Casarett and Doull's toxicology, 3rd ed., New York, MacMillan Publishing Company, p.29.

112. LAMB, J.C. & CHAPIN, R.E. (1985) Fertility assessment by continuous breeding. J. Am. Coll. Toxicol., 4: 173-184.

113. LEEMING, N.M., COZENS, D.D., & PALMER, A.K. (1987) Points for consideration in the design of multigeneration studies, Huntingdon, United Kingdom, Huntingdon Research Centre.

114. LEHMAN, A.J. & FITZHUGH, O.G. (1954) 100-fold margin of safety. Food Drug Off. US Q. Bull., 13: 51-58.

115. LOTTI, M., BECKER, C.E., & AMINOFF, M.J. (1984) Organophosphate polyneuropathy: pathogenesis and prevention. Neurology, 34: 658-662.

116. LU, F.C., JESSOP, D.C., & LAVALLE, A. (1965) Toxicity of pesticides in young versus adult rats. Food Cosmet. Toxicol., 3: 591-596.

117. LUSTER, M.I., DEAN, J.H., & MOORE, J.A. (1982) Evaluations of immune functions in toxicology. In: Hayes, W.A., ed. Principles and methods of toxicology, New York, Raven Press, pp. 561-586.

118. MACKENZIE, J.M., ZAKARIJA, M., & BONNYNS, M. (1979) Hyperthyroidism. Endocrinology, 1: 429-459.

119. MACKENZIE, W.F. & GARNER, F.M. (1973) Comparison of neoplasms in six sources of rats. J. Natl Cancer Inst., 50: 1243-1257.

120. MANSON, J.M. (1986) Teratogens. In: Klaassen, C.D., Amdur, M.O., & Doull, J., ed. Casarett and Doull's toxicology, 3rd ed., New York, MacMillan Publishing Company, pp. 195-222.

121. MIHICH, E. & KANTER, P.M. (1987) The toxicology of biological response modifiers. In: Berlin, A., Dean, J., Draper, M.H., Smith, E.M.B., & Spreafico, F., ed. Immunotoxicology, Hingham, Maryland, Martinus Nijhoff Publishers, pp. 208-218.

122. MURPHY, S.D., & CHEEVER, K.L. (1968) Effect of feeding insecticides. Inhibition of carboxyesterase and cholinesterase activities in rats. Arch. environ. Health, 17: 749-759.

123. NARAHASHI, T. (1982) Cellular and molecular mechanisms of action of insecticides: neurophysiological approach. Neurobehav. Toxicol. Teratol., 4: 753-758.

124. OECD (1981) OECD Test guidelines 1981. Report from the OECD Expert Groups on Short-term and Long-term Toxicity, Paris, Organization of Economic Cooperation and Development.

125. OECD (1983) OECD Guidelines for testing of chemicals. Section 4: Health effects, Paris, Organization for Economic Cooperation and Development (Guideline 416).

126. OFFICE OF SCIENCE AND TECHNOLOGY POLICY (1985) Chemical carcinogens: A review of the science and its associated principles. Fed. Reg., 49: 10371-10442, 50: 10372-10442.

127. PAGET, G.E. (1970) The design and interpretation of toxicity tests. In: Methods in toxicology, Oxford, London, Blackwell Scientific Publishers, pp. 1-10.

128. PALMER, A.K. (1981) Regulatory requirements for reproductive toxicology. In: Kimmel, C.A. & Buelke-Sam, J., ed. Developmental toxicology, New York, Raven Press, pp. 259-287.

129. PALMER, A.K. (1986) A simpler multigeneration study (poster presentation). In: Greenhalgh, R. & Robert, T.R., ed. Proceeding of the 6th IUPAC Congress on Pesticide Chemistry, 10-15 August, Oxford, Blackwell Scientific Publications.

130. PARKE, D.V. (1977) Biochemical aspects. In: Raven, R.W., ed. Principles of surgical oncology, New York, London, Plenum Medical Press, pp. 113-156.

131. PARKE, D.V. (1979) The role of the endoplasmic reticulum in carcinogenesis. In: Coulston, F., ed. Regulatory aspects of carcinogenesis and food additives: The Delaney Clause, New York, Academic Press, pp. 173-187.

132. PARKE, D.V. (1982) Survey of drugs-metabolizing enzymes. Biochem. Soc. Trans., 11: 457-548.

133. PARKE, D.V. & IOANNEDES, C.L. (1984) Reactive intermediates and oxygen toxicity in liver injury. In: Keppler, D., Popper, H., Bianchi, L., & Reutter, W., ed. Mechanisms of hepatocyte injury and death, Lancaster, MTP Press, pp. 37-48.

134. PARKE, D.V. & SYMONS, A.M. (1977) The biochemical pharmacology of mucus. In: Elstein, M. & Parke, D.V., ed. Mucus in health and diseases, New York, London, Plenum Medical Press, pp. 423-441.

135. PAYNTER, O.E. (1984) Oncogenic potential guidance for analysis and evaluation of long-term rodent studies, Washington, DC, US Environmental Protection Agency, Office of Pesticides and Toxic Substances (Evaluation Procedure No. 1000.1).

136. PAYNTER, O.E. & SCHMITT, R. (1979) The acceptable daily intake as a quantified expression of the acceptability of pesticide residues. In: Giessbuhler, H., ed. Advances in pesticide science, Oxford, Pergamon Press, pp. 674-679.

137. PAYNTER, O.E., BURIN, G.J., JAEGER, R.B., & GREGORIO, C.A. (1986) Neoplasia induced by inhibition of thyroid gland function (guidance for analysis and evaluation), Washington, DC, US Environmental Protection Agency, Standard Evaluation Procedure.

138. PAYNTER, O.E., BURIN, G.J., JAEGER, R.B., & GREGORIO, C.A. (1988) Goitrogens and thyroid follicular cell neoplasia: Evidence for a threshold process. Regul. Toxicol. Pharmacol., 8: 102-119.

139. PROBST, G.S. & HILL, L.E. (1987) Influence of age, sex and strain on the in vitro induction of unscheduled DNA synthesis in rat hepatocyte primary cultures. Cell Biol. Toxicol., 3: 113-126.

140. PURVES, H.D. & GRIESBACH, W.E. (1947) Studies on experimental goitre. VIII. Thyroid tumors in rats treated with thiourea. Br. J. exp. Pathol., 28: 46-53.

141. RIBELIN, W.E., ROLOFF, M.V., & HOUSER, R.M. (1984) Minimally functional rat adrenal medullary pheochromocytomas. Vet. Pathol., 21: 281-285.

142. ROE, F.J.C. & BAR, A. (1985) Enzootic and epizootic adrenal medullary proliferative disease of rats: influence of dietary factors which affect calcium absorption. Hum. Toxicol., 4: 27-52.

143. ROSIN, A. & UNGAR, H. (1957) Malignant tumors in the eyelids and the auricular region of thiourea-treated rats. Cancer Res., 17: 302-305.

144. SANTOLUCITO, J.A. & MORRISON, G. (1971) EEG of rhesus monkeys following prolonged low-level feeding of pesticides. Toxicol. appl. Pharmacol., 19: 147-154.

145. SCHALLER, R.T. & STEVENSON, J.K. (1966) Development of carcinoma of the thyroid in iodine-deficient mice. Cancer, 19: 1063-1080.

146. SEARLE, C.E. (1984) Chemical carcinogens, Washington, DC, American Chemical Society, Vol. 2 (ACS Monograph No. 182).

147. SENANAYAKE, N. & JOHNSON, M.K. (1982) Acute polyneuropathy after poisoning by an organophosphate insecticide. New Engl. J. Med., 306: 155-157.

148. SINHA, D., PASCAL, R., & FURTH, J. (1965) Transplantable thyroid carcinoma induced by thyrotropin. Arch. Pathol., 79: 192-198.

149. SRINIVASAN, V., MOUDGAL, N.R., & SHARMA, P.S. (1957) Studies on goitrogenic agents in food. I. Goitrogenic action of groundnut. J. Nutr., 61: 87-95.

150. STEVENS, K.R. & GALLO, M.A. (1986) Practical considerations in the conduct of chronic toxicity tests. In: Hayes, A.W., ed. Principles and methods of toxicology, New York, Raven Press, pp. 53-77.

151. SU, M., KINOSHITA, F.K., FRAWLEY, J.P., & DUBOIS, K.P. (1971) Comparative inhibition of aliesterases and cholinesterases in rats fed eighteen organophosphorus insecticides. Toxicol. appl. Pharmacol., 20: 241-249.

152. SUMI, N., STAVROV, D., FROHBERG, H., & JOCHMANN, G. (1976) The incidence of spontaneous tumors of the central nervous system of Wistar rats. Arch. Toxicol., 35: 1-13.

153. SWARM, R.L., ROBERTS, G.K.S., LEVY, A.C., & HINES, L.R. (1973) Observations of the thyroid gland in rats following the administration of sulfamethoxazole and trimethoprim. Toxicol. appl. Pharmacol., 24: 351-363.

154. TARONE, R.E. (1982) The use of historical control information in testing for a trend in proportions. Biometrics, 38: 215-220.

155. TASK FORCE OF PAST PRESIDENTS (1982) Animal data in hazard evaluation: Paths and pitfalls. Fundam. appl. Toxicol., 2: 101-107.

156. TAUROG, A. (1979) Hormone synthesis. Endocrinology, 1: 331-342.

157. THOMPSON, S.W. & HUNT, R.D. (1963) Spontaneous tumors in the Sprague-Dawley rat: Incidence rates of some types of neoplasms as determined by serial section versus single section technics. Ann. NY Acad. Sci., 108: 832-845.

158. TILSON, H.A. & CRANMER, J.M., ed (1985) Neurotoxicology in the fetus and the child. Proceedings of the 4th International Neurotoxicology Conference, Little Rock, Arkansas, 9-13 September 1985. Neurotoxicology, 7: 1-669.

159. US EPA (1982) Pesticide assessment guidelines. Subdivision F - Hazard evaluations: humans and domestic animals, Washington, DC, US Environmental Protection Agency, pp. 130-137.

160. US EPA (1983) Good laboratory practice standards: Toxicology testing. Fed. Reg., 48: 53922.

161. US FDA (1978) Good laboratory practice regulations. Fed. Reg., 43(274): 49986-60020.

162. US FDA (1982) Toxicological principles for the safety assessment of direct food additives and color additives used in food, Washington, DC, US Food and Drug Administration, National Toxicology Information Service, pp. 80-107.

163. VAN LEEUWEN, F.X.R., FRANKEN, M.A.M., & LAEBER, J.G. (1987) The endocrine system as the target in experimental toxicology. Adv. vet. Sci. comp. Med., 31: 121-149.

164. VETTORAZZI, G., ed. (1977) General principles in the toxicological evaluation of pesticide residues in food. In: Handbook of international food regulatory toxicology, Volume 1: Evaluations, New York, London, SP Medical and Scientific Books, pp. 93-142.

165. VOS, J.G. (1987) The role of histopathology assessment of immunotoxicity. In: Berlin, A., Dean, J., Draper, M.H., Smith, E.M.B., & Spreafico, F., ed. Immunotoxicology, Hingham, Maryland, Martinus Nijhoff Publishers, pp. 125-134.

166. VOUK, V.B. & SHEEHAN, P.J., ed. (1983) Methods for assessing the effects of chemicals on reproductive functions, New York, John Wiley and Sons.

167. WARD, J.M. (1983) Background data and variations in tumor rates of control rats and mice. Prog. exp. Tumor Res., 26: 241-258.

168. WARD, J.M. & RICE, J.M. (1982) Naturally occurring and chemically induced brain tumours of rats and mice in carcinogenesis bioassays. Ann. NY Acad. Sci., 26: 304-319.

169. WHO (1967) Procedures for investigating intentional and unintentional food additives. Report of a WHO Scientific Group, Geneva, World Health Organization (WHO Technical Report Series, No. 348).

170. WHO (1974) Assessment of the carcinogenicity and mutagenicity of chemicals. Report of a WHO Scientific Group, Geneva, World Health Organization (WHO Technical Report Series, No. 546).

171. WHO (1978) IPCS Environmental Health Criteria 6: Principles and methods for evaluating the toxicity of chemicals, Part 1, Geneva, World Health Organization.

172. WHO (1983a) Report of a Strategy Meeting on Updating Principles of Methodology for Testing and Assessing Chemicals in Food, Oxford, United Kingdom, 19-25 September, Geneva, World Health Organization (ICS(Food)/83) (Unpublished report).

173. WHO (1983b) IPCS Environmental Health Criteria 27: Guidelines on studies in environmental epidemiology, Geneva, World Health Organization.

174. WHO (1984) IPCS Environmental Health Criteria 30: Principles for evaluating health risks to progeny associated with exposure to chemicals during pregnancy, Geneva, World Health Organization.

175. WHO (1986) IPCS Environmental Health Criteria 60: Principles and methods for the assessment of neurotoxicity associated with exposure to chemicals, Geneva, World Health Organization.

176. WHO (1987) IPCS Environmental Health Criteria 70: Principles for the safety assessment of food additives and contaminants in food, Geneva, World Health Organization.

177. WHO (1989) Guidelines for predicting dietary intake of pesticide residues, Geneva, World Health Organization.

178. WILLIAMS, G.M. & WEISBURGER, J.H. (1986) Chemical carcinogens. In: Klaassen, C.D., Amdur, M.O., & Doull, J., ed. Casarett and Doull's Toxicology, 3rd ed. New York, MacMillan Publishing Company, pp. 99-173.

179. WOO, D.C. & HOAR, R.M. (1972) "Apparent hydronephrosis" as a normal aspect of renal development in late gestation of rats: the effect of methyl salicylate. Teratology, 6: 191-196.

180. WOO, Y., LAI, D.Y., ARCOS, J.C., & ARGUS, M.F. (1985) Chemical induction of cancer - Structural bases and biological mechanisms, New York, Academic Press, Inc., pp. 357-394.

181. ZBINDEN, L.C. (1987) A toxicologist's view of immunotoxicology. In: Berlin, A., Dean, J., Draper, M.H., Smith, E.M.B., & Spreafico, F., ed. Immunotoxicology, Hingham, Maryland, Martinus Nijhoff Publishers, pp. 1-11.

182. FAO/WHO (1965b) Evaluation of the toxicity of pesticide residues in food. Report of the Second Joint Meeting of the FAO Committee on Pesticides in Agriculture and the WHO Expert Committee on Pesticide Residues, Geneva, World Health Organization (FAO Meeting Report No. PL/1965/10/1; WHO/Food Add./27.65).

183. FAO/WHO (in press) Pesticide residues in food - 1989. Report of the Joint Meeting of the FAO Working Party of Experts on Pesticide Residues and the WHO Expert Committee on Pesticide Residues, Rome, Food and Agriculture Organization of the United Nations.

ANNEX I. GLOSSARY

I. 1 Abbreviations Used in this Document

ADI Acceptable Daily Intake

CEC Commission of the European Communities

CNS Central Nervous System

FAO Food and Agriculture Organization of the United Nations

GLP Good Laboratory Practice

IARC International Agency for Research on Cancer

IPCS International Programme on Chemical Safety

JECFA Joint FAO/WHO Expert Committee on Food Additives

JMPR Joint FAO/WHO Meeting on Pesticide Residues

LD_{01} Lethal Dose, 1%

LD_{50} Lethal Dose, median

MRL Maximum Residue Level

MTD Maximum Tolerated Dose

NCI National Cancer Institute (USA)

NOAEL No-Observed-Adverse-Effect Level

NOEL No-Observed-Effect Level

NTE Neurotoxic Esterase

NTP National Toxicology Program (USA)

OECD Organization for Economic Cooperation and Development

OP Organophosphate

SAR Structure/Activity Relationship

TADI Temporary Acceptable Daily Intake

TH   Thyroid Hormone

TOCP   Tri-*O*-Cresyl Phosphate

VSD   Virtually Safe Dose

TSH   Thyrotropin

WHO   World Health Organization

I. 2 Definitions of Terms Used in this Document

Acceptable Daily Intake (ADI): An estimate by JMPR of the amount of a pesticide, expressed on a body weight basis, that can be ingested daily over a lifetime without appreciable health risk (standard man = 60 kg).

Codex Alimentarius Commission: The Commission was formed in 1962 to implement the Joint FAO/WHO Food Standards Programme. The Commission is an intergovernmental body made up of more than 130 Member Nations, the delegates of whom represent their own countries. The Commission's work of harmonizing food standards is carried out through various committees, one of which is the Codex Committee on Pesticide Residues. JMPR serves as the advisory body to the Codex Alimentarius Commission on all scientific matters concerning pesticide residues.

Effect: A biological change in an organism, organ, or tissue.

Elimination (in metabolism): The expelling of a substance or other material from the body (or a defined part thereof), usually by a process of extrusion or exclusion, but sometimes through metabolic transformation.

Embryo/fetotoxicity: Any toxic effect on the conceptus resulting from prenatal exposure, including structural or functional abnormalities or postnatal manifestation of such effects.

JMPR: JMPR is a technical committee of JMPR specialists acting in their individual capacities. Each is a separately-constituted committee, and when either the term "JMPR" or "the Meeting" is used, it is meant to imply the common policy or combined output of the separate Meetings over the years.

Long-term toxicity study: A study in which animals are observed during the whole life span (or the major part of the life span) and in which exposure to the test material takes place over the whole observation time or a substantial part thereof. The term chronic toxicity study is used sometimes as a synonym for "long-term toxicity study".

Lowest-observed-effect level (LOEL): The lowest dose of a substance which causes changes distinguishable from those observed in normal (control) animals.

No-observed-adverse-effect level (NOAEL): The highest dose of a substance at which no toxic effects are observed.

No-observed-effect level (NOEL): The highest dose of a substance which causes no changes distinguishable from those observed in normal (control) animals.

Safety factor: A factor applied by JMPR to the no-observed-effect level to derive an acceptable daily intake (the no-observed-adverse-effect level is divided by the safety factor to calculate the ADI). The value of the safety factor depends on the nature of the toxic effect, and the quality of the toxicological information available.

Short-term toxicity study: An animal study (sometimes called a sub-acute or subchronic study) in which the effects produced by the test material, when administered in repeated doses (or continuously in food or drinking-water) over a period of about 90 days, are studied.

Temporary ADI: Used by JMPR as an administrative procedure to permit the continued acceptance of the pesticide pending submission of new toxicological data.

Teratogen: An agent which, when administered prenatally, induces permanent abnormalities in structure.

Teratogenicity: The property (or potential) to produce structural malformations or defects in an embryo or fetus.

Threshold dose: The dose at which an effect just begins to occur, that is, at a dose immediately below the threshold dose the effect will not occur, and immediately above the threshold dose the effect will occur. For a given chemical there can be multiple threshold doses, in essence one for each definable effect. For a given effect there may be different threshold doses in different individuals. Further, the same individual may vary from time to time as to his or her threshold dose for any effect. However, given the present state in the development of science, for certain chemicals and certain toxic effects, a threshold dose may not be demonstrable.

The threshold dose will fall between the experimentally determined no-observed-effect level (NOEL) and the lowest-observed-effect level (LOEL). Of importance is that when using the NOEL or LOEL, it should be specified which effect is being measured, in what population, and what is the route of administration. In situations for which the effect of concern is considered to be adverse, the terminology often used is that of a no-observed-adverse-effect level (NOAEL) or lowest-observed-adverse-effect level (LOAEL), again specifying the effect, the population, and the route of administration. Both the NOEL and LOEL (as well as the NOAEL and LOAEL) have been used by different scientific groups as a surrogate for the threshold dose in the performance of risk assessments.

Toxicity: The toxicity of a compound is its potential to cause injury (adverse reaction) to a living organism.

ANNEX II. APPROXIMATE RELATION OF PARTS PER MILLION IN THE DIET TO MG/KG BODY WEIGHT PER DAY[a]

Animal	Weight (kg)	Food consumed per day (g) (liquids omitted)	Type of diet	1 ppm in food = (mg/kg body weight per day)	1 mg/kg body weight per day = (ppm of diet)
Mouse	0.02	3		0.150	7
Chick	0.40	50		0.125	8
Rat (young)	0.10	10	Dry laboratory chow diets	0.100	10
Rat (old)	0.40	20		0.050	20
Guinea-pig	0.75	30		0.040	25
Rabbit	2.0	60		0.030	33
Dog	10.0	250		0.025	40
Cat	2	100		0.050	20
Monkey	5	250	Moist, semi-solid diets	0.050	20
Dog	10	750		0.075	13
Man	60	1500		0.025	40
Pig or sheep	60	2400		0.040	25
Cow (maintenance)	500	7500	Relatively dry grain forage mixtures	0.015	65
Cow (fattening)	500	15 000		0.030	33
Horse	500	10 000		0.020	50

[a] Lehman, A.J. (1954) *Association of Food and Drug Officials Quarterly Bulletin*, **18**: 66. The values in this table are average figures, derived from numerous sources.

Example: What is the value in ppm and mg/kg body weight per day of 0.5% substance X mixed in the diet of a rat?

Solution: I.   0.5% corresponds to 5000 ppm.

II. From the table, 1 ppm in the diet of a rat is equivalent to 0.050 mg/kg body weight per day. Consequently, 5000 ppm is equivalent to 250 mg/kg body weight per day (5000 x 0.050).

INDEX

Absorption, 17, 28, 31, 32, 37, 71, 72, 73, 74, 75
Acetylcholinesterase inhibition, 63, 64
Acute studies, 17
ADI
    conditional, 82
    temporary, 16, 17, 25, 26, 48, 77, 78, 81, 82, 85
Autolysis, 39, 40, 46

Behavioural toxicity, 14
Biochemical studies, 17, 54
Bioengineered organisms, 86
Biological half-life, 17
Biomarkers, 76
Biorational products, 86
Bipyridilium compounds, 88
Body weights, 46

Carbamates, 30, 45, 63, 64, 65, 67
Carboxylesterases, 87
Carcinogenic pesticides, 52
Carcinogenicity
    classification schemes, 51, 52
    genotoxic, 67, 68
    limited evidence of, 48
    organophosphates, 88
    principles, 53
    studies, 15, 17, 20, 31, 32, 47, 50, 80
    testing, 47, 88
Clearance, 75
Clinical chemistry, 36, 43, 44, 45, 46
Codex Committee on Pesticide Residues, 85
Commonly occurring tumours, 49
Comparative metabolic data, 29, 52, 73, 75, 76
Comparative pharmacokinetic data, 20, 59, 73, 75, 76

Delayed neurotoxicity, 18, 61, 62, 63, 67
Dietary intakes, 50, 83
Dose/response
    and safety factors, 79
    from accidental poisonings, 28
    in carcinogenicity, 51, 52
    in delayed neuropathy, 62, 67

in human volunteers, 27
relationships, 19, 29, 41

Electron microscopic examination, 40
Enterohepatic circulation, 72
Environmental Health Criteria, 29, 49, 50, 51
Epidemiological studies, 29

FAO, 13, 15, 17, 21, 22, 27, 30, 53, 80, 84
Food intake, 46, 47, 50, 56

Goitrogenic carcinogens, 88
Good Laboratory Practices (GLP), 25, 26

Haematological examinations, 35, 44
Half-life, 17, 75, 81
Histopathological examinations, 39, 40, 46, 47
Historical control data, 34, 40, 41, 42
Human
       Cell lines, 33
       Volunteers, 27, 29

Immunotoxicity, 14, 68, 69, 70
Impurities, 21, 22, 23, 87
In utero, 57, 58
In vitro, 27, 28, 33, 37, 64, 68
In vivo, 27, 28, 29, 33, 37, 45, 49, 60, 64, 65, 68, 70, 88
Industrial Bio-Test Laboratories, 26
Inert ingredients, 23
Ingested dose, 47
Intermediates, 21
International Agency for Research on Cancer (IARC), 35
IPCS, 13, 58, 70
Isomers, 22, 23, 62, 63

JECFA, 13, 31, 71, 77

Lactation, 54, 55, 56, 57, 58
LD_{01}, 36
LD_{50}, 18, 31, 33, 36, 63, 66

Long-term studies
    and ADI, 15, 18, 32, 80
    and reproduction, 56, 58
    conduct of, 31, 34, 38, 39, 43, 73
    interpretation of, 20, 37, 72

Maternal toxicity, 54, 59
Maximum Tolerated Dose (MTD), 37
Mechanisms of toxicity, 20, 73
Metabolites
    (animal), 28, 31, 36-37, 44, 53, 57, 69, 71-74
    (plant), 81
Michaelis-Menten kinetics, 74
Mixtures, 23, 62, 63, 84
Mouse liver tumours, 49, 50
MRLs, 13, 16, 17
Mutagenicity, 32, 67, 68

Neuropathy target esterase (NTE), 62
Neurotoxicity, 17, 18, 30, 61, 62, 63, 65, 66, 67
Nitrosamines, 30
No-observed-adverse-effect-level (NOAEL), 17-18, 20, 23, 42, 46-47, 52, 76-79, 82, 87, 90

Occupational exposure, 27, 28
Oncogenes, 49
Ophthalmological effects, 87
Organophosphates, 45, 62, 67, 87, 88

Peroxisome proliferation, 32
Pharmacokinetic data, 73, 76
Plasma cholinesterase, 19, 64, 67
Poison Control Centres, 27
Proprietary data, 25
Protein binding, 37, 72
Pyrethroids, 22, 65, 66

Radioactive labelling techniques, 75
Re-evaluation of pesticides, 85
Reproduction
    and ADI, 18, 82
    dose response, 19
    follow-up studies, 55

maternally toxic doses, 37
(multigeneration) study, 17, 22, 53, 54, 56-61, 82
Routes of exposure, 14, 48, 74

Safety factors
and ADI, 17, 77, 78, 79, 83
and TADI, 82,
determination of, 42, 77, 78, 79, 80
in absence of toxicity, 18
in carcinogenicity, 52
Satellite groups, 51
Screening teratology studies, 60
Short-term studies, 18, 31, 34, 36, 45
Special stains, 40
Sperm measurements, 58
Stability, 21, 22, 23, 47, 75
Statistical analysis, 36, 51
Structure-activity relationships, 17, 30, 88

Task Force of Past Presidents of the Society of Toxicology, 41
Technical grade, 21, 22, 23
Teratogenicity, 17, 18, 57, 58, 60, 82
Tetrachloro-dibenzo-p-dioxin (TCDD), 21
Threshold, 18, 20, 63, 79, 90
Thyroid
Hormone, 89, 90
Neoplasia, 90
Tolerance, 16
Tumours
benign, 51
malignant, 20, 51

Urinalysis, 35, 43, 44

Validity of data, 25

www.ingramcontent.com/pod-product-compliance
Lightning Source LLC
Chambersburg PA
CBHW071713210326
41597CB00017B/2470